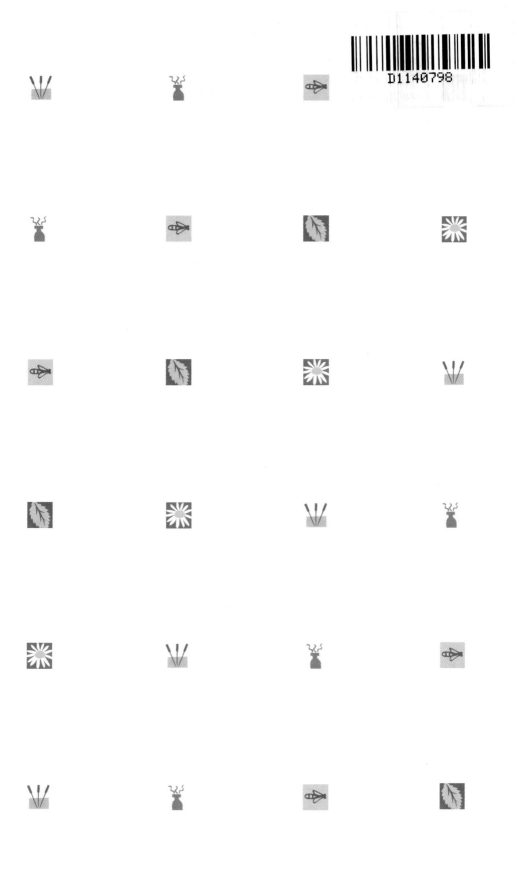

Heal Your

DOG

The Natural Way

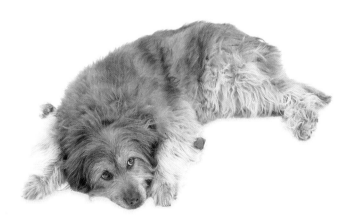

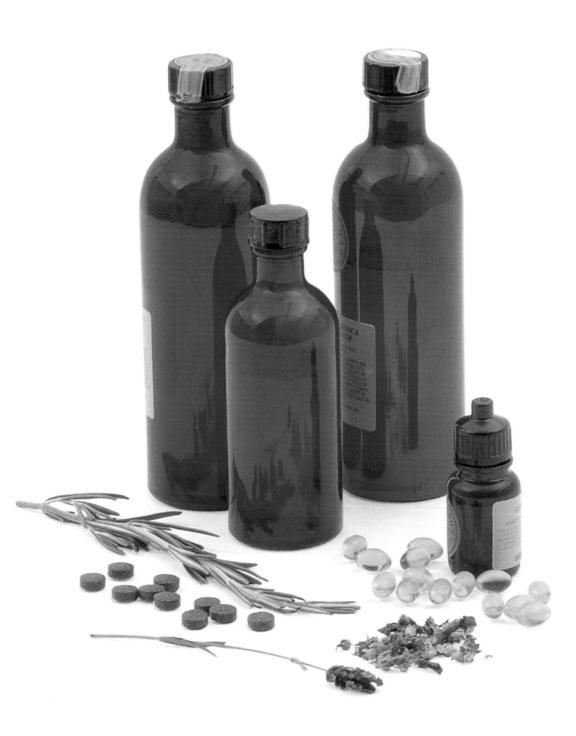

Heal Your
DOG
The Natural Way

RICHARD ALLPORT

For Maggie:

> *'I fear darkness, I fear night*
> *Don't leave me empty of your light'*

With thanks to Susan Lee for typing
an intelligible manuscript from my
illegible handwriting.

Senior art editor: Luise Roberts
Commissioning editor: Samantha Ward-Dutton
Project editor: Jane Royston
Copy editors: Cathy Lowne, Claire Musters
Designer: Tony Truscott
Photography: Jane Burton
Picture research: Liz Fowler
Production: Rachel Lynch

First published in Great Britain in 1997 by Mitchell Beazley,
an imprint of Reed Consumer Books Limited, Michelin House,
81 Fulham Road, London SW3 6RB and Auckland, Melbourne,
Singapore and Toronto.

ISBN 1 85732 811 6

A CIP catalogue of this book is available at the British Library.

Printed in Hong Kong

contents

6 introduction

8 natural therapies
10 aromatherapy
13 homoeopathy
17 herbal medicine
21 Bach flowers
24 acupuncture
28 minor therapies
38 a healthy life

50 common diseases
and conditions
52 emergencies
60 skin
66 ears and eyes
73 respiratory system
76 cardiovascular system
80 endocrine system
83 musculo-skeletal system
91 nervous system
94 digestive system
103 urinary system
106 female reproductive system
111 male reproductive system
113 cancer
115 parasites
118 specific infections
120 behaviour

126 appendix: list of abbreviated
homoeopathic terms

126 acknowledgements

127 index

introduction

As modern medicine increases in complexity, as scientific knowledge grows more all-encompassing and as technology becomes more high-powered, can there still be a place for the old remedies in the treatment of disease? With so many new drugs and a multitude of revolutionary techniques available, what need can there be for the healing power of herbs, for the holistic approach of homoeopathy, or for the ancient art of acupuncture?

There are many disadvantages to the use of drugs in conventional medicine. New drugs often need to be produced because diseases have developed a resistance to their predecessors, and these are inordinately expensive to research, produce, test and license. Side-effects from their use are ever-present, and the new drugs often simply do not work effectively. Arthritis, eczema, disease of the immune system and colitis (inflammation of the colon) are just a handful of the common diseases that still remain incurable as far as modern medicine is concerned.

It is no wonder that there has been a change in our attitudes to the traditional remedies. No longer are they dismissed as folklore and old wives' tales, as all over the world we are rediscovering the health-giving, healing powers of therapies that have for centuries been safe and effective. The very fact that herbal treatments, homoeopathy and acupuncture, along with numerous other therapies, are currently enjoying a resurgence is a tribute to our growing awareness that natural medicines have a great deal to offer.

Many people would agree with these sentiments so far. But for dogs? Can acupuncture cure an Afghan, or homoeopathy help a husky? The answer is yes. This book aims to show how natural medicines are as applicable to our canine friends as they are to us, by explaining which medicines and therapies are beneficial for which conditions, and by outlining in simple terms the best approaches to their use. Another great advantage of natural therapies is that, although some treatments (such as acupuncture) must be carried out by a qualified practitioner, many other techniques are simple to learn and can be undertaken by any dog owner at home, with little effort or expense. Indeed, some treatments – such as aromatherapy massage with fragrant essential oils – may be a pleasurable experience for owner and dog alike!

All you will need in order to find this book of practical help is an open mind, an interest in health – and, of course, a dog.

important note

Before starting to use this book, please do remember one vital point: it is NOT intended to be a substitute for seeking professional veterinary assistance for your dog whenever necessary. Never try to diagnose and treat illness solely from the information in these pages. If you are ever in any doubt about your dog's health or welfare, you must consult your vet – remember that failure to do so could put your dog's life at risk.

using this book
The first section, *natural therapies*, explores the five main therapies commonly used to treat dogs – aromatherapy, homoeopathy, herbal medicine, Bach flowers and acupuncture – and then looks at various lesser-used, 'minor' therapies. With the main therapies, information is given on their origins and development, on what kind of problems should respond to them, and on how the medicines should be used to achieve the best results. A case history to illustrate the effectiveness of each therapy is included. There is also a short description of each minor therapy, with advice on its application. It is important to follow the instructions carefully, as natural remedies are not automatically completely safe – in aromatherapy, essential oils given by mouth can be toxic if given too frequently; a homoeopathic remedy in the wrong potency can aggravate symptoms.

Advice is then given on how providing a suitable environment, well-chosen foods and natural supplements can help to keep a cat healthy and accelerate recovery from illness. Potential drawbacks of commercial cat foods are discussed, and there is a guide to feeding a home-made diet. Many natural medicines are available in tablet form, and this section ends with tips on giving tablets quickly and efficiently.

The *natural therapies* section should be used in conjunction with *common diseases and conditions* to ensure that the right therapy is administered in the correct way. In this second section, many of the common illnesses suffered by dogs, and the natural remedies that can be used to relieve the symptoms, are covered. It is ordered by body systems and their ailments: for example, remedies for arthritis will be found within the musculo-skeletal system. Case studies throughout reveal the remarkable results that natural medicines can achieve.

natural

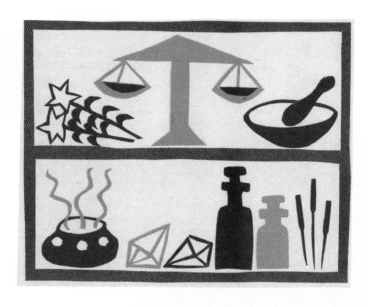

therapies

An old saying in medicine declares that there is 'a pill for every ill', and there is certainly no shortage of healing therapies for dogs. The aim that is common to all the natural medicines is to restore balance and equilibrium to the body – a case perhaps of 'a remedy to restore order to every disorder'.

None of the therapies included here will have any adverse effect on conventional drugs, but you should keep your vet informed of any natural remedies that you use. Unfortunately, some conventional drugs do interfere with the effectiveness of natural medicines: homoeopathic remedies and biochemical tissue salts in particular are rendered less effective by steroids and some hormones. However, essential oils, herbal medicine, and flower and gem essences normally work very well alongside conventional drugs.

Most natural therapies are compatible with each other, and it is quite acceptable and often very beneficial to use more than one at a time. The only drawback here is that it can be dificult to assess which therapy is creating the greatest improvement. There are some exceptions: for example, homoeopathic remedies and biochemical tissue salts may be adversely affected by aromatic essential oils and by strong-smelling herbs (especially Garlic); similarly, it would not be wise to follow a session of osteopathy too closely with physiotherapy treatment. However, in general, all the natural therapies are compatible and complementary. When administered in the correct dosages, natural medicines are also very safe.

All the medicines suggested should produce an obvious improvement in symptoms within the time stated. If any remedy administered in the dosage advised has no effect after a normal course, you should choose a different remedy. Of course, if your dog is suffering from an acute problem that does not respond to treatment, you must consult your vet as soon as possible.

aromatherapy

Aromatherapy involves the use of essential oils derived from plants as a treatment for a range of illnesses. Although used for centuries in human ailments, aromatherapy for dogs is a fairly recent phenomenon.

The essential aromatic oils are obtained by a distillation process, and the resulting product is a highly concentrated oil, with – as the name implies – a strong fragrance. Each oil has its own individual properties when used as a therapeutic remedy. However, in general, essential oils are antiseptic and detoxifying, and also help to strengthen the immune system and to regulate the metabolism. The exact mode of action is not yet understood but, as with all natural therapies, it seems that it is the energy within the oil that interacts with the energy in the patient to produce the healing effect.

Just some of the beneficial responses to aromatherapy include the painkilling action of Lavender and Marjoram; the anti-arthritic effect of Juniper, Pine and Sandalwood; improvement in digestive problems following the use of Caraway and Coriander; and the relief of respiratory symptoms with Eucalyptus and Thyme.

treatment

There are three main ways to administer essential oils: by mouth (oral administration), by massage and by diffusion.

oral administration

Oils can be given by mouth, but this is a method that should only be undertaken with the strict supervision of an expert in aromatherapy techniques. This is because essential oils are so concentrated that even small amounts can have a toxic effect.

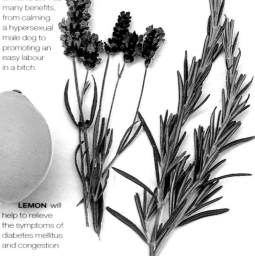

ROSEMARY is a widely used herb that is especially useful in relieving arthritic stiffness and revitalizing a dog suffering from a serious condition such as cancer

LAVENDER has many benefits, from calming a hypersexual male dog to promoting an easy labour in a bitch

LEMON will help to relieve the symptoms of diabetes mellitus and congestion

A wide range of plants, fruits and herbs is used to make fragrant aromatherapy oils, each of which has its own unique properties.

massage

This method is the one that is most commonly used. One drop of the appropriate oil is added to 2.5 ml (½ tsp) of an inert 'carrier' oil such as Wheatgerm, Sweet-almond or Sunflower. The role of a carrier is to dilute the essential oil, allowing it to be absorbed through the skin. A few drops of the diluted mixture is massaged into a hairless – or the least-hairy – area of skin (usually the 'armpit' area, the groin, or an inner thigh). Three to four minutes of gentle massage will allow sufficient oil to be absorbed.

In general, an aromatherapist will recommend twice-daily massage for five days as a typical dosage regime. Neat essential oils must never be applied directly to the skin, as in this concentrated form they can result in rashes and soreness.

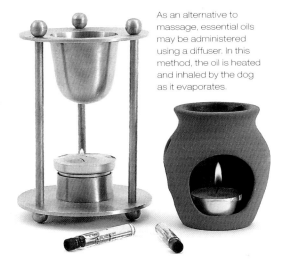

As an alternative to massage, essential oils may be administered using a diffuser. In this method, the oil is heated and inhaled by the dog as it evaporates.

diffusion

In this technique a diffuser is used to evaporate the oil, which is then inhaled by the patient. The diffuser should be left in operation with the dog in the same room for about 30 minutes so that sufficient oil is absorbed. This procedure will generally need to be repeated twice daily for five days. Diffusers are relatively inexpensive to buy, and come with simple setting-up instructions.

suitability

Aromatherapy has a rapid action – a few days' treatment is normally all that is required – and the fragrant remedies are very pleasant to use. They are also readily available: health-food stores, pharmacies and even beauty-product outlets stock or can obtain essential oils. Do ensure, however, that the oils are of true plant origin rather than being synthetic (this information should be given on the product label), as the latter appear to be less effective.

The disadvantages involve administering the oils to dogs. As has been discussed, oral dosing is not normally advisable, while massage can be a problem: most dogs do seem to appreciate a gentle massage for a few minutes each day, but some quickly become bored and can be difficult to keep still. Diffusers are straightforward to use, but can be messy and are also fairly time-consuming.

One further drawback of aromatherapy is the cost: essential oils are expensive, and have only a limited shelf-life, particularly if purchased already diluted in a carrier oil. It would certainly be prohibitively expensive to keep a stock of all the essential oils mentioned in this book. Simply buy the oils as you need them.

Another option is to locate an aromatherapist who has experience of using essential oils for animals, and to ask your vet to refer your dog when the need arises. This will also ensure that the correct diagnosis is made, and that both you and the aromatherapist know exactly what condition is being treated. In this way you can be certain that the essential oils used will be just right for your dog.

As in the case study below, there are many instances where a health problem seems to have been eliminated by conventional drugs, when they have in fact 'pushed' the problem back into the body, only for it surface later in another form. Natural medicines are much more likely to push the problem out of the body and allow a permanent cure.

aromatherapy case study

Vera was an Afghan hound who was afflicted by chronic sinusitis (see page 74). She had previously suffered from a bout of 'kennel cough' (see page 118) after spending two weeks in boarding kennels, and this had been treated with a course of antibiotics. Although the persistent coughing caused by the virus had stopped, Vera developed an annoying catarrh in the sinuses, which additional treatment with antibiotics failed to clear up.

Vera's owner happened to be an aromatherapist and, after coming into my surgery to discuss the dog's symptoms, set up a diffuser using a blend of Eucalyptus, Pine and Thyme essential oils. Vera seemed to enjoy settling down for a 30-minute session of inhalation twice a day, and, within five days, her sinusitis had cleared and she could breathe easily again.

Apart from demonstrating how successful aromatherapy can be, this case also illustrates how conventional drugs can sometimes suppress disease while allowing a chronic condition to develop.

homoeopathy

In the late 18th century doctors were probably killing as many patients as they cured, bloodletting was still practised, and many 'medicines' were actually poisons. However, at this time a German doctor, Samuel Hahnemann, developed a medical system – based on lengthy observation and rigorous experimentation – that he called homoeopathy. Today, it is an irony that homoeopathy is derided as unscientific by some members of the medical establishment, when in fact it was founded purely on scientific principles in an age of quackery in medicine.

Hahnemann found that a substance of mineral, plant or animal origin that causes adverse symptoms in an individual could cure those same symptoms when given in a minute, 'energized' homoeopathic dose. For example, Arsenic caused severe gastro-enteritis if swallowed, but homoeopathic Arsenic would actually cure the symptoms of the condition.

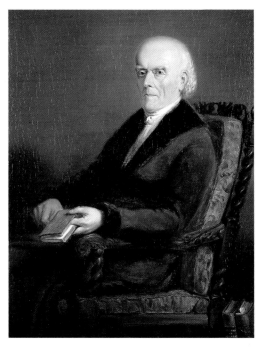

The German physician, Dr Samuel Hahnemann (1755–1843): the founder of homoeopathy.

Homoeopathic remedies are produced by diluting the original substance in several stages, and by shaking, or 'succussing', the solution at each dilution to add energy to the product. This system of increasingly diluting but also energizing the starting material results in remedies that are so dilute as to be completely safe and free from side-effects, yet are powerful enough to act as strong healing agents.

Remedies are made from a number of minerals, including Arsenic, Phosphorus and Lead; from plants such as Belladonna, Aconite and Arnica; and from animal products ranging from the honeybee (Apis mellifica, commonly known as Apis mel.) to the venom of poisonous snakes (such as Lachesis). There are currently over 3000 different homoeopathic remedies in use, all working on Hahnemann's principle that 'like cures like', and that a remedy given in a small dose will cure the symptoms caused by the material substance.

Hahnemann also discovered that his homoeopathic remedies corresponded to the mental and emotional state of a patient. So, for example, the kind of individual who would benefit from homoeopathic Arsenic tended to be anxious and restless, to seek comfort and warmth, to drink small amounts of fluids frequently, and to dislike cold, wet weather. On the other hand, a lazy, overweight and relaxed character, who lived to eat, drink and sleep would suit homoeopathic Calcarea Carbonica (Calc. Carb.).

This idea of a homoeopathic 'constitution' – that is, the concept that each individual person (or animal) is a physical, mental and emotional type and will correspond to a particular homoeopathic remedy – is especially useful when dealing with chronic and deepseated disease. Homoeopathy can be used to treat almost all diseases found in dogs, but is especially effective for chronic conditions such as skin disorders, arthritis and colitis (inflammation of the lining of the colon).

Homoeopathic remedies are commonly known by abbreviations of their Latin names, and have been listed as such in the *common diseases and conditions* section of this book. The full names of the remedies may be found on page 126.

treatment

Homoeopathic remedies are available as tablets, powders, granules (pillules), liquids and ointments. Tablets are the most widely available form, and the dosage rates quoted in this book are applicable to these, which are as follows:

acute conditions

Give one tablet every 15 minutes for three hours, then one tablet hourly for the rest of the day. After this, give one tablet three times daily for three further days, or until all symptoms have disappeared.

chronic conditions

Give one tablet three times daily for one week, followed by one tablet twice daily for three weeks.

If other forms of remedy are used, the equivalent doses are as follows: One tablet = one powder = 12 granules = three drops of liquid.

Remedies are also produced in different potencies. The commonly available potency is known as 6c, and this will be marked on the tablet container. The correct remedy for a condition will be effective in any potency, but the higher the potency (the larger the number before the 'c') the greater the healing action will be. However, if too high a potency is given the symptoms may temporarily become aggravated, so use 6c potencies only (unless advised otherwise by a vet).

Homoeopathic remedies should be given directly by mouth, if possible (for the correct technique on giving tablets to dogs, refer to page 49). This should be done away from food and without touching the tablets, to avoid the risk of contamination: the effectiveness of these medicines can be reduced by certain chemicals in foodstuffs and even by traces of chemicals on fingers. (Herbs with powerful aromas – such as Garlic – may also reduce the potency of homoeopathic remedies, and so should not be given at the same time.) It is usually possible to shake a tablet from the container into the cap, and then to drop it from the cap into the dog's mouth (or into a special syringe: see page 49).

Some manufacturers produce soft tablets that dissolve in the mouth within a few seconds; however, most tablets on the market are hard and take a little longer to be absorbed. As homoeopathic tablets are absorbed better through the mouth lining than through the stomach after being swallowed, it may be preferable to crush a hard tablet into a powder first, in a folded sheet of clean paper. The paper can then be made into a 'funnel' to tip the powder into the dog's mouth. If a dog is wary of taking tablets, a remedy may be coated with a little butter. However, homoeopathic tablets should not be mixed with a large quantity of food, as the effectiveness of absorption may be reduced. Nor, ideally, should they be given within 30 minutes of a meal.

On many containers you will see instructions such as 'two tablets for an adult, one for a child'. In fact, as a homoeopathic preparation is giving the body an energy input rather than a physical substance, the dose is the same for all animals (including humans) of any size. There is not twice the effect when giving two tablets, and a single tablet is all that is ever necessary at one time. The only reason that manufacturers put this instruction on the label is because they believe that we expect an adult to take a larger dose than a child!

storing homoeopathic remedies

Remedies must be stored away from odours, bright light and excessive heat or cold. Magnetic fields from electrical equipment can also make them less effective. Although this makes homoeopathic products sound fragile, if stored correctly they remain active for years.

homoeopathy case study

Dexter was a two-year-old English springer spaniel in desperate trouble. He was suffering from an unusual form of arthritis that can affect young dogs, and was almost crippled as a result. Despite visits to a veterinary orthopaedic specialist, his condition had been pronounced incurable, and Dexter seemed destined to a life of pain, stiffness and constant drug therapy. His owner brought him to me for homoeopathic treatment as a last resort, before deciding whether to have him put to sleep.

Apart from the bone and joint damage caused by his disease, Dexter was as bright and bouncy as it was possible to be. His owner informed me that he had been a very lively, active dog, that he loved attention, was nervous of sudden noises, had always been thin and lightweight, and was rather prone to vomiting shortly after eating.

This and other information convinced me that Dexter would respond to the homoeopathic remedy Phosphorus. This suits animals with the physique and the behavioural characteristics shown by Dexter, and is also an appropriate remedy for bone and joint damage. Taken in a material dose, Phosphorus causes bone decay and degeneration (this was seen many years ago in girls employed to put Phosphorus heads on matches: their jaw bones degenerated as a result of inhaled Phosphorus fumes). In homoeopathic terms, the remedy made from Phosphorus – on the principle that 'like cures like' – will therefore help in bone and joint disease. Soon after starting a course of homoeopathic Phosphorus Dexter was much improved, and within a few weeks was running around as though he had never been stiff at all. An occasional short course of this remedy is enough to keep him mobile, pain-free and active.

Some months later, Dexter's owner telephoned to tell me that Dexter had cut his tongue several days earlier, and that the wound was still bleeding. I suggested an extra course of Phosphorus, because it is also a good remedy for wounds that will not heal, or that continue bleeding. This was successful, and the bleeding stopped rapidly and completely, and did not recur.

This case history shows how one homoeopathic remedy can be used to treat more than one condition or disease, as well as the importance of taking a holistic approach rather than simply considering the physical symptoms of illness.

herbal medicine

Herbal medicine, or phytotherapy as it is more correctly known, is probably the oldest system of natural medicine used by humans. Nothing could be more natural than harnessing the healing powers of the herbs and flowers around us to cure our diseases and those of our pets; indeed, animals in the wild have an uncanny ability to seek out plants to help them when they are ill.

Modern drugs may be isolated herb extracts or synthetic derivatives of these substances. Aspirin (from willow tree bark) and Digitalis (from the foxglove) have herbal origins and are still widely used today. However, isolated extracts and synthetic compounds are more likely to cause side-effects, and have less overall healing power than the herbs themselves. Herbal medicines are gentler and safer, but no less effective than their conventional counterparts.

Herbal medicine aims not only to treat symptoms, but to restore normal bodily functions so that natural healing can occur. Over 2000 medicinal plants are used today, many of which have been revered for their healing properties since ancient times.

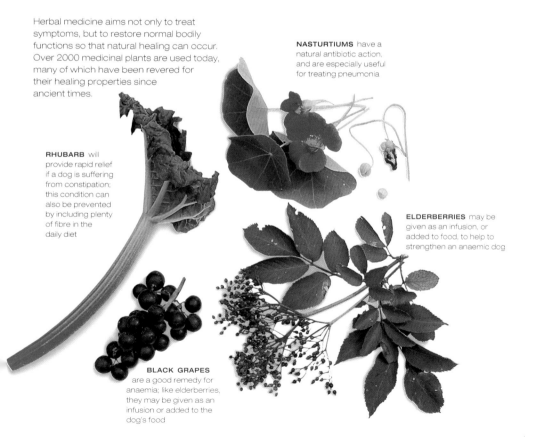

NASTURTIUMS have a natural antibiotic action, and are especially useful for treating pneumonia

RHUBARB will provide rapid relief if a dog is suffering from constipation; this condition can also be prevented by including plenty of fibre in the daily diet

ELDERBERRIES may be given as an infusion, or added to food, to help to strengthen an anaemic dog

BLACK GRAPES are a good remedy for anaemia; like elderberries, they may be given as an infusion or added to the dog's food

treatment

Herbal remedies may be obtained from herbalist shops, or can be prepared at home from wild plants – such as Nettles and Dandelions.

proprietary herbal remedies

Many commercially prepared remedies are now available for dogs, usually in tablet form. This makes dosing easier, as tablets are often more acceptable to dogs than infusions (see below). Tinctures and lotions are also widely available, and are easy to administer. For all such products, be sure to follow the instructions on the packaging precisely, and take care not to overdose.

infusions

Some herbs are not yet available in the 'user-friendly' forms of tablets, tinctures or lotions. The standard way to administer a herb of this type is by infusion: simply take 1 tsp of the dried herb, pour on a cup of boiling water and leave to stand for 20 minutes. Strain and allow to cool, and the mixture is ready.

An infusion will remain active for several days if kept cool, but many herbalists recommend making up a fresh mixture every two days. For an acute condition, give the infusion twice daily with food for one week, in the following amounts:

up to 9 kg (20 lb) body weight –
    15ml (3 tsps)
9–23 kg (20–50 lb) body weight –
    20 ml (4 tsps)
23–36 kg (50–80 lb) body weight –
    25 ml (5 tsps)
36 kg (80 lb) upwards –
    30 ml (6 tsps)
For a chronic condition, use the same dosage rate but continue for eight to 12 weeks.

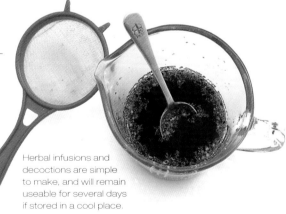

Herbal infusions and decoctions are simple to make, and will remain useable for several days if stored in a cool place.

decoctions

Add herbs consisting of bark, roots or other hard tissue to boiling water, at the ratio of 15 ml (3 tsps) per 300 ml (½ pt) of water. Boil for 20 minutes, then strain and allow to cool. Administer as for an infusion.

If you gather your own herbs, it is important to ensure that they have not been sprayed with pesticides. Use the freshly picked herbs on the same day, or air-dry them before use in a well-ventilated room (the herbs should well-separated for drying, not bunched together). Once dried, herbs have a fairly long shelf-life, but should ideally be used within 12 months.

suitability

Herbal remedies are particularly effective for chronic problems. For instance, Skullcap with Valerian is helpful for persistent hyperactive behaviour, and Slippery elm for ongoing digestive disorders. If given correctly, the advantages of the gentle action and the history of known effectiveness of herbal therapy make it an ideal treatment for many conditions. All the herbs in the *common diseases and conditions* section can be used safely in the dosage rates specified here.

However, some lesser-used herbs can be difficult to obtain, and preparing and administering infusions or decoctions can be time-consuming. A dog's response to herbal medicines can also be slow: it may take up to two weeks before you see any improvement, and you may need to continue for a few months for maximum benefit.

More importantly, there is a risk of giving too little or too much: an overdose of some herbal remedies can be fatal. If you wish to use herbal medicines, always choose those sold for dogs, and administer them according to directions or on the advice of an experienced vet.

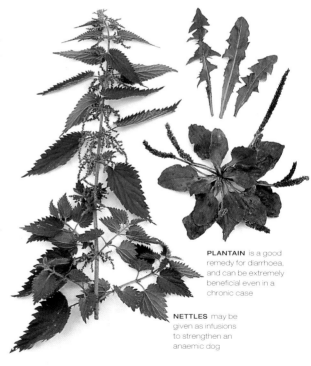

DANDELION will help to relieve the symptoms of a range of diseases, including arthritis, liver disease and recurrent cystitis; it may also promote hair growth in a case of alopecia

PLANTAIN is a good remedy for diarrhoea, and can be extremely beneficial even in a chronic case

NETTLES may be given as infusions to strengthen an anaemic dog

Many herbs are common and readily available, but rare varieties should only be obtained from herbalists.

herbal-medicine case study

Holly and Ivy were two fully grown yellow labradors, sisters from the same litter, who lived happy, healthy lives together. Unfortunately, whenever the temperature began to rise in the summer months, both dogs would develop sudden and fairly severe bouts of diarrhoea. First Holly would suffer a bout, and then Ivy would follow suit. By the time Ivy's problem had started to settle down, it would be Holly's turn to start up again.

Despite extensive investigations, no cause for the diarrhoea could be found: no bacteria or virus seemed to be responsible, and no sudden dietary alterations or other changes in lifestyle had been made. As soon as the weather cooled again at the end of the summer, the diarrhoea always vanished mysteriously. This syndrome of summer diarrhoea is not uncommon in dogs, but for both sisters to suffer was unfortunate – and exasperating for their owner. Various conventional treatments had had very little effect: antibiotics and antidiarrhoeal compounds would suppress one incident of diarrhoea, but not prevent the next one from occurring.

The difficulty was solved by the herb Bilberry, whose berries can be dried and used to produce a potent antidiarrhoeal remedy (the berries are fairly hard and 'woody', so the herbal medicine is made as a decoction rather than an infusion – see page 18).

Holly and Ivy were given 20 ml (4 tsps) of the decoction twice daily. Within two weeks their diarrhoea had ceased, and during what became a long, hot summer only one episode of diarrhoea recurred. After four weeks the dosage was reduced to once daily, and after another four weeks to dosing on alternate days. The following year, at the first sign of hot weather, dosage with the same decoction recommenced: this was given twice daily for two weeks, once daily for two weeks, and then on alternate days for the rest of the summer. This pattern has been repeated for several years, with almost total success.

One important word of warning. When they are fresh, Bilberries have quite the opposite effect to the dried berries, as the fruit acid present in fresh berries, together with an irritant action of the pips, produces a laxative effect. If your dog is suffering from a bout of constipation, by all means give freshly picked Bilberries, but for diarrhoea dried berries are essential!

Bach flowers

The Bach flower essences are named after Dr Edward Bach, a highly respected bacteriologist and homoeopath who worked for many years at the Royal London Homoeopathic Hospital. He subsequently turned his attention to the healing powers of flowers, plants and trees, and – first in Wales and later in Oxfordshire – immersed himself in studying their potential for resolving mental and emotional problems. Dr Bach was convinced that physical illness and mental states are closely linked and that, by stabilizing and balancing any mental or spiritual problems, physical disease would be cured as a follow-on process.

Dr Bach developed a process of 'energizing' the healing potential of the energy within flowers. He found that the action of sunlight on the petals (or other parts) of chosen plants that were floated in water would transfer the healing energy from the plant into the water. He added a few drops of this energized water to brandy, which acted as a preservative, and the resulting mixture was Bach flower essence.

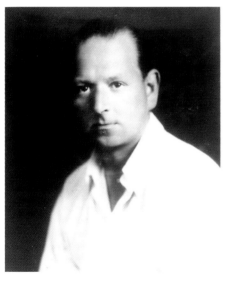

Dr Edward Bach developed his range of flower essences to treat a range of emotional and behavioural problems, which he considered to be linked to physical disease.

In all, Dr Bach produced 38 different flower essences, each of which has a specific effect on mental, emotional or behavioural problems. For instance, Aspen is beneficial for anxiety, vague fears and apprehensions; Impatiens is used to treat feelings of irritability, impatience and over-reaction; Mimulus is helpful for specific fears such as fear of noise or of the dark, as well as for general shyness and timidity; and Vine is the source of a remedy that can overcome strong feelings of dominance and a need for power. If a physical illness seems to be linked with a mental or emotional problem, the therapy will almost certainly relieve the symptoms of the physical disease as well.

In addition to the 38 single remedies, a further Bach flower product was developed from a mixture of five of the original essences, and its components have a remarkable effect in cases of shock, collapse and trauma. The combination is known as Rescue Remedy, and is probably the best-known of the Bach flower range.

treatment

Depending on the ailment, it is quite common when using Bach flower essences to give more than one remedy at a time. The remedies should be administered as follows.

Bach flowers

The essences can be administered directly by mouth (see opposite). Alternatively, they may be added to drinking water or to a small amount of food. When taken by humans, the remedy is normally diluted, and then four drops given four times daily. Dogs seem to respond better to the 'neat' essence, given as one drop twice daily. The treatment should be continued for four to eight weeks in order to achieve the full effect.

Rescue Remedy

This should be used at times of accident and trauma. In this case, give one drop every five minutes for one hour, or until a change to other treatment is made.

tablets

Bach flowers are also available in the form of proprietary tablets; refer to the instructions on the container for dosage. (For the technique of giving tablets, see page 49.)

suitability

Bach flower remedies are readily available (most health-food stores stock or can obtain them), and the range is small and straightforward. It is usually easier to select one of 38 Bach flowers than one of over 3000 homoeopathic remedies, or over 2000 medicinal plants used in herbal medicine! The flower essences are simple to administer (drops are often easier to give than tablets when dosing dogs).

Disadvantages of using Bach flowers are that the therapy is restricted to problems associated with behaviour or the emotions, and that it is vitally important to understand a dog's state of mind in order to be able to use Bach flowers effectively. Treatment is generally fairly long-term (there are no side-effects, so this is perfectly safe): dosage for four to eight weeks is necessary in most cases to obtain the full effect. When the desired result has been achieved, therapy can often be discontinued, but in some cases it may be required indefinitely to maintain the improvement.

giving Bach flower essence

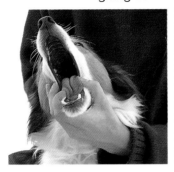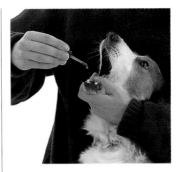

1 Draw up the essence into the dropper, then hold the dog's head and gently tilt it backwards so that the lower jaw begins to drop. Still holding the head with one hand, use the thumb and fingers of the other hand to hold down the lower jaw.

2 Pick up the dropper, and hold it over the dog's open mouth (taking care not to touch the mouth as you do this, to avoid contamination of the dropper). Administer the drop or drops, aiming towards the back of the tongue, then release the dog's head.

Bach flowers case study

Layla was a West Highland white terrier who had always been a little nervous and highly-strung. Her owners had recently moved house, to a noisier area. Layla had hated the move, refused to settle at her new home, and spent most of each day trembling in her basket, apparently full of anxiety, as well as resentment. Her owners were sure that Layla blamed them entirely for her unhappiness, and that she was 'taking it out' on them.

Several remedies were indicated here: Walnut for difficulty in adjusting to a change in life, Wild rose for apathy and lack of interest, and Willow for resentment and a 'poor me' attitude. These three essences, along with Mimulus for the very noticeable fear of noise, produced a profound change for the better in Layla. Within a few days she was brighter, began to be affectionate towards her owners again, and was eventually persuaded to go out for walks. The remedies were given daily for four weeks and then twice weekly for a further four weeks, after which time Layla was – to her owners' great relief – her old self once again.

acupuncture

Acupuncture is the ancient Chinese art of inserting needles at selected points in the body. It has a venerable history, with treatment recorded as many as 3000 years ago.

The traditional Chinese belief is that energy flows freely through the body along specific channels, or meridians, and that disease is the result of an imbalance or blockage in this energy flow. By inserting fine needles at precise points along the meridians, the energy flow can be stimulated, sedated or balanced, and, in this way, the healing process will begin to take place.

This theory is the starting point for the successful treatment of a whole range of diseases. Acupuncture can be employed as a therapy for almost any condition, but is particularly helpful for problems in the musculo-skeletal system – such as arthritis (see pages 83–4), back pain, and ligament and tendon injuries (see page 85), and in the nervous system (including trapped nerves, paralysis and chronic degenerative radiculo myelopathy: see page 89).

Acupuncture is probably best-known for its effectiveness in helping to relieve pain, but it is much more than simply an unusual form of painkiller. Some other important functions include healing damaged tissue, helping to regenerate nerves and stimulating the immune system, and these are just some of the many ways in which this therapy can be a powerful agent for treating illness in dogs.

treatment

Acupuncture therapy must only be carried out by a vet trained in the technique: never attempt to use acupuncture needles yourself at home. Acupuncture therapy usually involves weekly sessions to begin with. Once improvement has occurred, sessions may graduate to four-weekly (or longer) intervals if continuing treatment is necessary. In most cases a significant response is seen within three sessions; if no improvement is noticeable after this, it is unlikely that further acupuncture will be of benefit.

Treatment will vary from, for instance, a dog with a sprained shoulder requiring six needles inserted once a week for three or four weeks – resulting in a lasting cure – to an old dog with chronic spinal arthritis, requiring 12 needles inserted once a week for six weeks, then once a month for six months, followed by a 'booster' session every two or three months for life. A cure is not expected for this kind of problem, but acupuncture is neverthless an important form of treatment as it will control the pain and stiffness.

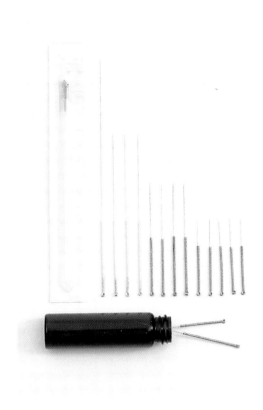

As a rule, dogs will accept the insertion of acupuncture needles surprisingly well. Most vets using this therapy find that only a tiny percentage of their patients really resent the needling procedure. Indeed, the vast majority of dogs will become relaxed and tranquil during sessions, and may even drop off to sleep.

Once the needles are in place, they will be quite painless provided that the patient remains still, although dogs who do try to move about may experience minor discomfort.

electro-acupuncture
With this technique, electrodes are attached to the needles and a small electric current then passes through the needles into the acupuncture point on the dog's body. This is said to amplify the healing effect.

Acupuncture needles are sterile and are used only once. Treatment is normally quite painless, and most dogs will tolerate the procedure quite happily.

moxibustion
Here, the dried Chinese herb, Moxa, is burned, and the resulting heat is applied either directly to the needle, or to the skin over the acupuncture point. The heat generated in this way is thought to enhance the healing effect, and the Chinese believe that Moxa itself is a herb with healing properties.

laser treatment
A more modern form of acupuncture involves focusing a laser beam on the acupuncture point. This has the advantage of being painless, but the disadvantage of requiring the use of expensive equipment. In most dogs, simple needling is perfectly sufficient, and the other forms of acupuncture tend to be used in those few cases where needles on their own are not producing the desired response.

suitability

The benefits of acupuncture include the rapid painkilling effect in many conditions, and the fact that between sessions no tablets or other treatments are required to maintain the effect. As the needles are sterile and used only once, there is no health risk. The only possible 'side-effect' is that a few dogs experience a temporary aggravation of symptoms. This 'getting worse before getting better' is a common syndrome among many of the natural therapies. It is not a true side-effect when compared with those associated with conventional drugs – it is simply a natural reaction of the body as it begins to throw off the disease.

The disadvantages are few: mainly the fact that the occasional dog is frightened or anxious when needles are inserted, and also that regular sessions are necessary. If the nearest vet practising acupuncture is some distance away, the travelling involved can be a negative factor for the owner.

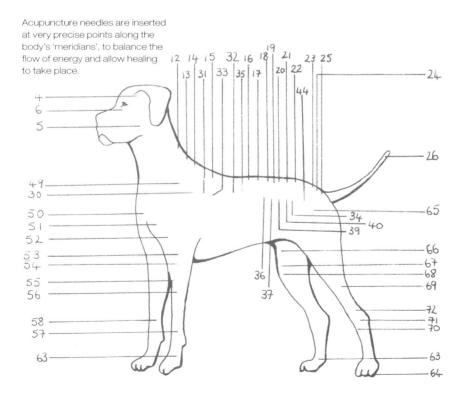

Acupuncture needles are inserted at very precise points along the body's 'meridians', to balance the flow of energy and allow healing to take place.

acupuncture case study

Storm was a five-year-old border collie with a history of auto-immune disease. This is a condition in which the body's immune system appears to become confused and, instead of attacking foreign invaders such as bacteria and viruses, begins to attack its own body tissues. Storm suffered from a particular form of auto-immune disease that resulted in general weakness, anaemia (a lack of red blood cells in the body – see pages 78–9) and also extensive skin damage. He had lost a great deal of his fur, and looked like a threadbare mop-head.

Despite intensive investigations and treatment with a range of conventional drugs, Storm's progress had so far been minimal. However, his owner had herself undergone acupuncture treatment in the past, and she was very interested to find out whether it could possibly help her dog.

Treatment began, using six needles per session. The points needled included Kaohuangshu (a point for debility after prolonged illness) and Housanli (a point used as a 'tonic' and for prevention of disease). There are hundreds of different acupuncture points on the body, some of which tend to be used more frequently and have specific names such as these. Storm was also given 100 mg of royal jelly daily (this supplement seems to have a stabilizing effect on some of the body's metabolic processes, especially those linked to coat condition and energy), as well an evening-primrose-oil supplement to improve the condition of his skin.

Within the first three sessions a visible improvement was apparent. Storm had considerably more energy, he was physically stronger, and his fur began to regrow. After six sessions of acupuncture at weekly intervals, he moved on to sessions at four-weekly and then at eight-weekly intervals. After 18 months of treatment, he was looking almost normal. He had regained the weight that he had lost, and his fur – although still a little on the thin side – was quite respectable. His anaemia had gone, and he was behaving as a healthy energetic border collie should do.

This case illustrates that acupuncture is not only useful for joint, spinal or nerve problems, but can also effectively treat other conditions. It also demonstrates that, with a chronic complaint, it can take time for symptoms to fade completely.

minor therapies

In addition to the main therapies described so far, there is a wide range of other natural therapies that may be used in the treatment of disease in dogs. Most are included in the following list, and are therapies that I have used on my canine patients, with varying degrees of success. There are a few other treatments that are not described here: these have been omitted either because I have no personal experience of their use, or have not sufficient evidence that dogs would respond to them.

biochemical tissue salts

Biochemical tissue salts were the discovery of a German doctor called William Schuessler. His theory was that, for body tissue to function in the best way, the cells must have a healthy balance of the 12 mineral salts that form a large part of the cells' composition. The minerals used are 'energized' as in homoeopathy, but only to a low potency; the energized mineral remedy (or a combination of several remedies) is then used as a treatment for a wide variety of conditions. Schuessler, by trial and experiment, discovered which tissue salts would be effective for which diseases.

Biochemical tissue therapy is by nature similar to homoeopathy, and can be used to treat a wide range of diseases. In general, tissue salts are very effective in the treatment of physical disease but, as there are only 12 remedies in the range compared with the thousands of homoeopathic remedies, the effects are often less specific.

The 12 tissue salts are commonly known by abbreviations of their Latin names, and have been listed as such throughout the *common diseases and conditions* section of this book. The salts are as follows: Calcarea fluorica (Calc. fluor.), Calcarea phosphorica (Calc. phos.), Calcarea sulphurica (calc. sulph.), Ferrum phosphoricum (Ferr. phos.), Kali muriaticum (Kali mur.), Kali phosphoricum (Kali phos.), Kali sulphuricum (Kali sulph.), Magnesia phosphorica (Mag. phos.), Natrum muriaticum (Nat. mur.), Natrum phosphoricum (Nat. phos.), Natrum sulphuricum (Nat. sulph.) and Silica (not abbreviated).

treatment

As biochemical tissue salts are produced in a similar way to homoeopathic remedies, and are available in tablet form, the dosage instructions are exactly the same as for homoeopathic preparations (see pages 14–15; see also page 49 for the correct technique of administering tablets to a dog).

Chinese medicine

Traditional oriental medicine has three main strands: herbal medicine (see pages 17–20), acupuncture (see pages 24–7) and food cures. The approach is a holistic one, so a practitioner may well use a combination of all three therapies.

The Chinese version of herbal medicine is somewhat different from the Western equivalent. Chinese phytotherapy involves the use of many different herbs, fungi and even shells, simmered for a long period with water until a concentrated liquid remains.

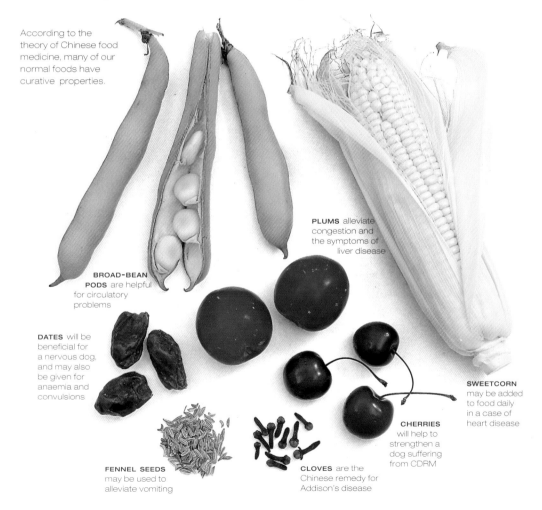

According to the theory of Chinese food medicine, many of our normal foods have curative properties.

PLUMS alleviate congestion and the symptoms of liver disease

BROAD-BEAN PODS are helpful for circulatory problems

DATES will be beneficial for a nervous dog, and may also be given for anaemia and convulsions

SWEETCORN may be added to food daily in a case of heart disease

CHERRIES will help to strengthen a dog suffering from CDRM

FENNEL SEEDS may be used to alleviate vomiting

CLOVES are the Chinese remedy for Addison's disease

In the dietary field, Chinese medicine views foods as treatments for disease. In general terms, pungent foods (such as ginger and onion) are warming and promote energy circulation. Sweet foods (such as honey and sugar) neutralize the toxic effects of other foods, and slow down acute symptom development. Sour foods (such as lemons and plums) are helpful for diarrhoea. Bitter foods (such as hops and radishes) reduce fever, but have a laxative effect. Salty foods (such as kelp and seaweed) soften hardened tissue, thus relieving muscle spasm and treating enlarged lymph glands.

treatment

Dogs may not be suitable patients for a total application of Chinese medicine, as the concentrated liquid produced in phytotherapy is invariably foul-tasting, and I have yet to meet a dog who would accept it. However, the same principles do apply as for humans, and a modified treatment using acupuncture, Western herbal medicine and a sprinkling of Chinese food cures where applicable is certainly an option. (For acupuncture methods, see pages 24–7; Chinese food cures are included where applicable in *common diseases and conditions*, along with their dosages and methods of administration.)

flower therapies

As well as Bach flower remedies (see pages 21–3), other lesser known but very effective flower essences are available. For instance, the Bailey flower essences are excellent, as are the Australian and Alaskan essences. There is even a Hawaiian aloha flower-essence range!

All these essences act, as do the Bach flowers, primarily at the level of the emotional and mental state of the patient. They therefore have a particular relevance for behavioural problems, or for a dog who is experiencing grief following the loss of a friend (canine or human), or distress and unhappiness in a boarding kennel.

treatment

Dosage rates for all these flower essences are as for Bach flower remedies (see pages 22–3).

T-touch massage

This is a type of massage developed by Linda Tellington-Jones, and is derived from the human massage and movement technique of Moshe Feldenkrais. The Tellington T-touch is a system of gentle, repeated massaging movements, which are said to generate specific brainwave patterns in the patient. The massage is especially beneficial for dogs suffering from anxieties, especially following injuries or surgery. It helps a dog to quieten and become calm, and then allows healing to take place more rapidly, so that the healing is both mental and physical.

treatment

The basic T-touch massage is a series of small, circular massage movements, as if pushing the fingers around a clockface, starting at six and pushing the skin slowly clockwise all the way round, past six again and finishing at eight. These massage circles are performed randomly all over the body and are continued for about 15 minutes. This procedure is repeated two or three times per day.

Massage sessions of 15 minutes should be given three times a day for a week in acute conditions, and for four weeks in chronic disorders.

reflexology

This is a way of treating disease in body organs by applying pressure to particular points, and its use was known in India and China as many as 5000 years ago. An American doctor, W. T. Fitzgerald, was the founder of modern reflexology. He found that, by applying pressure to his (human) patients' hands, he could relieve pain. This technique was developed by Eunice Ingham into the better-known foot reflexology.

Although the anatomy of a dog's foot is different from our own, the principles of reflexology hold good for our animal companions, and some reflexologists are beginning to work with animals.

treatment

The theory that certain areas of the feet and hands correspond to certain organs and glands in the body is related to the theory of the acupuncture meridians, almost all of which end in the hands and feet (or, in the case of a dog, all four feet). Applying pressure at points in the feet is akin to stimulating 'end-of-meridian' points in acupuncture. Reflexology is based on the same principle of unblocking energy flows, and the response to treatment is usually broadly similar.

colour therapy

To many people's surprise, colour can be used to treat disease. Each colour in the spectrum has an effect on physical and mental well-being, and has its own energy that can interact with a patient in a positive way.

For instance, red helps to increase energy levels (in the form of red clothing, it has been shown to increase blood pressure in a person), and will help in treating diseases such as circulatory problems and asthma. Conversely, blue is calming and reduces blood pressure, and will assist in the treatment of conditions as epilepsy and diarrhoea. Orange might be used for anaemia and phobias; yellow for eczema and arthritis. Green is balancing, and will help heart problems and emotional trauma. Indigo is the colour for ear and eye disease, while violet is a relaxing colour, effective for kidney disease and sinusitis.

treatment

The obvious argument against the use of colour therapy for dogs is that they do not see in colour, but it is not necessary to see the colour to derive benefit from it. This is because it is the energy of the colour that is absorbed by the body – not the ability to visualize it – that is important, making colour therapy perfectly applicable to dogs.

From the simple expedient of encouraging a dull, depressed dog to lie on a red blanket, to classic colour therapy in which coloured light is focused on the patient, colour can be a beneficial therapy. If you are using colour yourself, expose your dog to the relevant colour – for instance, by resting on a coloured blanket – for up to two hours a day.

A colour therapist, or chromopractitioner, may also be willing to work with animals, on referral from a vet; in this case, he or she will advise on the sessions required.

crystals and gems

The first recorded use of crystals and gems as healing agents can be traced back to Ancient Egypt. All crystals and gems, and indeed humans and dogs, vibrate at their own frequency, and the interaction between the energy field of the canine patient and that of the crystal will allow a stabilizing and healing action to occur. All crystals and gems have different healing properties. Amethyst, for example, is a potent pain reliever (for physical and emotional pain). Ruby is beneficial for arthritic symptoms,

The energy field of crystals and gems interacts with and acts to stabilize the energy field of the patient, allowing natural healing to occur. The crystal or gem being used should be placed near the relevant 'chakra', or energy centre, of the body.

Emerald for colitis (inflammation of the lining of the colon), and Citrine quartz will help to heal tissue damage after accidents and trauma.

how to administer

If visiting a crystal therapist after referral from a vet, full instructions will be given. If using crystals yourself, you can attach them to the dog's collar or harness, which should be worn for two to three hours a day. Alternatively, place them on or around the body: they work particularly well at the traditional energy centres (chakras) of the body, such as at the top of the head, the throat and the stomach area. The crystals should be left in place for up to two hours a day.

In electro-crystal therapy, a sealed tube of crystals is placed on the affected part of the body (or on the related energy centre). The crystals are activated by an electrical current, and work by stabilizing energy imbalances.

An alternative method of gem therapy is the use of liquid remedies. These are liquefied drops of crystals, minerals and gemstones, and are administered as for Bach flower essences (see page 22), with one drop given once or twice daily by mouth or in drinking water. Like Bach flowers, gem remedies are particularly applicable to mental and emotional disorders. For example, Sapphire is helpful for hyperactivity and anxiety, while Onyx might be used for the dominant, aggressive dog.

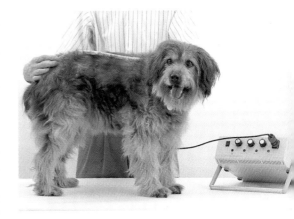

electro-crystal therapy

Electro-crystal therapy (ECT) is a technique that was pioneered by the scientist Harry Oldfield, and is used to diagnose and treat any energy imbalances that may occur in the body. It harnesses the known healing effect of crystals, and works according to the same basic principles, but amplifies the effect by the use of electricity.

In this therapy, quartz crystals, placed in saline solution in a sealed tube, are stimulated by a small electric current at high frequency. The energy field created by the crystals under this stimulation interacts with the energy field of the patient, and stabilizes energy imbalances. This allows healing of a wide range of illnesses, from bronchitis to back pain. The tube contains different crystals, and varying frequencies of the electric current stimulates particular crystal types, enhancing the healing action of the crystals that vibrate at those frequencies.

treatment

Treatment involves placing a sealed tube of crystals on the affected area (or on the energy centre that is linked with that area) and then setting the appropriate frequency on a small generator connected to the tube. Sessions normally last for between 10 and 20 minutes, depending on the severity of the problem. There is no discomfort while treatment is taking place, and no risk to the patient.

Sessions are usually given at weekly intervals initially, and may then be reduced to longer intervals as an improvement in the ailment becomes apparent. Some qualified electro-crystal therapists are prepared to treat dogs, on referral from a vet.

healing

In a sense, healing – often known as spiritual or faith healing – is the purest form of treatment for illness, as it involves no pills, needles or equipment of any kind. The laying on of hands to heal disease is of ancient origin, and in all societies and cultures people with healing powers are acknowledged.

The source of the healing power is a matter of debate. Some healers believe that their abilities are divinely inspired, others claim to have 'spirit guides', while some may have no fixed ideas about the derivation of the powers. However, all healers seem to feel that they act as a channel for the healing energy, rather than doing the healing themselves. One particular form of hands-on healing, called Reiki, was developed by Mikao Usui, a Japanese theologian, who discovered in ancient Sanskrit writings a method of laying on hands that is now practised and taught worldwide.

Most reputable healers (in the UK) belong to the National Federation of Spiritual Healers, which operates in a strictly ethical and professional manner. The Federation has a code of conduct specifically regarding the treatment of animals. This was drawn up in conjunction with the Royal College of Veterinary Surgeons, and is an important guide to which all its members adhere.

Healing can be effective with any illness or problem from which dogs suffer, including mental and behavioural disorders as well as physical conditions. It has also often been shown to be of great benefit for 'incurable' diseases such as cancer and liver disease. Even if a complete cure is not achieved, animals almost always seem to feel better after healing sessions, with an apparent reduction in their level of pain or discomfort.

treatment

Healing sessions consist of a period of 10 to 20 minutes on average, during which the hands of the healer are held on or above the problem area. Many human patients report feeling a warm sensation in that part of the body. We obviously do not know whether dogs feel the same effect, but most remain quiet and content during sessions. The number and frequency of healing sessions needed to help a patient will depend on the severity of the condition, but once a week until the condition is cured or under control is normal.

iridology

As with dowsing, iridology is primarily a diagnostic technique rather than a therapy. The colour and shape of the iris, and its various marks, flecks and discolorations reveal to the practised observer a mass of information regarding present health status, the location and type of any disease present, and any tendency towards future disease.

treatment

Different areas of the iris correspond to different parts of the body. Through careful examination of each eye under magnification, an iridologist will attempt to assess the exact location of the disorder, or where it may occur. The idea of this is to determine the root cause of the problem, so that it can be treated.

physiotherapy

Especially well-known for its undoubted ability to restore the use of damaged muscles, ligaments, tendons and bones, physiotherapy involves a range of techniques. There is in the UK an Association of Chartered Physiotherapists in Animal Therapy whose members are skilled in the treatment of pets, and many dogs have benefited from their expert attention.

treatment

The most common form of treatment involves manipulation of the affected body parts. Other techniques may include using ultrasound, laser beams and even short-wave diathermy (a method of warming the muscles to accelerate the healing process).

The therapist to whom your dog is referred will suggest a schedule for treatment sessions, normally starting on a weekly basis. The total duration of treatment will depend on progress of the disorder.

osteopathy

This is a manipulative therapy that has been practised for over 100 years. Although particularly effective for spinal problems in dogs, osteopathy can also be used for disorders of the joints and muscles. To the lay person, osteopathy and chiropractic (see below) have much in common and may seem indistinguishable, but these two schools of manipulative therapy maintain that their techniques are quite separate.

As far as the canine patient is concerned, both osteopathy and chiropractic have proven invaluable in the case of chronic back problems and persistent joint, muscle and nerve conditions. A number of osteopaths are willing to treat animals on referral from a vet, and many dogs are a testament to their undoubted skills.

treatment

Osteopathy involves manipulation of the affected body parts. The therapist to whom your dog is referred will suggest a schedule for treatment sessions, normally starting on a weekly basis. The duration of treatment will depend on progress of the disorder. In some instances one or two sessions of manipulation are sufficient; in other cases a longer course of treatment is necessary.

chiropractic

Chiropractic is a manipulative therapy that is used to treat muscular and joint disorders, especially those of the spine.

Although chiropractic was developed as a therapy for humans, and the anatomy of the dog is different from our own, the technique can be successfully applied to problems such as lameness and joint injuries. Some chiropractors will treat dogs, on referral from a vet.

treatment

Chiropractors use conventional investigative techniques – such as X-ray pictures – to diagnose problems. Manual stretching and massage are used to reduce muscle spasm and to ease joint stiffness. The chiropractor will advise on the length and frequency of treatment sessions. On average, three to 10 weekly sessions are required.

radionics

This is another natural therapy that is based on the energy pattern created by an individual, and on the belief that a disruption in this pattern is a reflection of the disease process. Radionics is a method of identifying any change in the body's energy pattern, and of finding ways of correcting it.

Dogs appear to respond well to radionics, and some practitioners of this therapy are beginning to specialize in treating them. A radionic practitioner may also recommend additional complementary therapies such as homoeopathy, osteopathy or physiotherapy.

treatment

A practitioner of radionics will take a clump of fur, or another small part of body tissue, from the dog: this is often known as the 'witness'. (On the principle that all parts of the body will reflect the energy disruption, a small sample of fur will be quite sufficient for a detailed analysis to be made.) The sample is scanned by a radionic instrument, which measures energy patterns and isolates the problem area in the body. Other radionic instruments are then used to 'broadcast' healing energy back to the patient, in order to correct the imbalance and stimulate healing to occur.

A radionics practitioner can operate at some distance from the patient, and, because treatment takes place via the 'witness', does not necessarily even need to see him or her. However, a full history of the illness, together with background information about any previous medical problems, and a general description, will be required.

The duration of a course of radionics treatment will vary according to the type of problem and the dog concerned. A recently acquired illness may improve within a few days; a chronic problem may take weeks or months to resolve.

dowsing

Rather more of a diagnostic tool than a therapy, it is interesting to note that the age-old art of dowsing has an ancient application in medicine. Although most of us have heard about and probably seen the art of dowsing for water, it is less commonly known that dowsing can be used to discover sites of disease in the body, and even to learn which remedy or remedies will be curative for that disease.

treatment

By noting the swing or oscillation of a pendulum (rather than using a forked twig) over a patient, an expert dowser can find out much information that may be useful in assessing the type and extent of disease, and the therapy that may be indicated.

a healthy life

This section is dedicated to the principle that prevention is better than cure. It concentrates on measures that can be taken to keep a dog fit and well, including the external factors that affect health, what a dog should be fed and what supplements will be beneficial when added to the canine diet.

your dog's environment

The main reason for any general improvement in health in all human societies is usually due to a better quality of living standards: clean drinking water, efficient sewage disposal, adequate ventilation, better hygiene, less-crowded living conditions and a good diet. These factors, far more than any modern medicines, reduce the risks of disease and allow us to live longer.

A safe, healthy environment is equally important for our dogs, in whom there appears to have been a marked increase in chronic conditions such as disease of the immune system, eczema and colitis. One reason for this may be the increasing pollution of the environment: of the air, of water, and of the land. The continuing overuse of chemicals on farmland, and the factory waste pumped into rivers and the air, are placing a burden both on our immune systems and on those of our dogs, particularly those prone to a chronic illness. However, taking the following measures may help to reduce the potential dangers in the environment, both outdoors and indoors.

air

Do not expose a dog with any degree of respiratory disease to cigarette smoke. Adequate ventilation at all times is also vital: this is another reason why dogs must never be left in cars on warm days. A dog with a history of coughs or other respiratory symptoms may benefit from the use of an ionizer to keep the air fresh and clean. A humidifier may also be worth considering if the air is very dry (for example, when central heating is in operation), as dry air is very harmful to the delicate respiratory-tract tissues.

Try to reduce the volume of any chemicals used around the house, such as fresh-air sprays, hair sprays and fly sprays, as these contain substances that may be harmful to a dog.

A humidifier is a simple device that is used to counter adverse effects of central heating and very dry air. A bowl of water placed near radiators will help to maintain moisture levels.

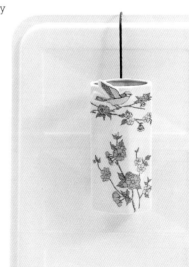

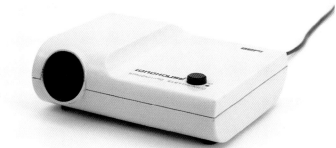

Ionizers can be expensive, but are a worthwhile investment. They will help to keep the air fresh and clean, and can be extremely beneficial for a dog who is prone to respiratory problems.

Avoid walking a dog in or near fields that have been recently sprayed with chemicals. Some dogs seem to suffer from a syndrome similar to human hay fever, so reducing the time allowed outside on days with high pollen counts is also worthwhile.

water

I firmly believe that tap water can aggravate health problems in some dogs. The chemicals that our added to tap water – such as chlorine – as well as any pollutants that may be present, appear to act as a precipitating factor in the progression of eczema, colitis (inflammation of the bowel) and other inflammatory disorders. Dogs certainly seem to prefer – and to benefit from – the use of filtered or mineral water rather than ordinary tap water.

Drinking and feeding bowls should be ceramic or stainless steel, as the chemicals from plastic may leach out into water or food.

land

Try to avoid allowing a dog to walk in fields to which fertilizer or other chemicals have been recently applied. Skin irritation can result, as can itchiness after running through certain grasses in the springtime. In the winter, avoid exercising a dog on roads or pavements which have been gritted and salted, as exposure to treated roads can cause severe foot inflammation.

It is said that nomadic people, and the animals that travel with them, seldom suffer from chronic illness. One theory for this is that many of us, who stay in one place for long periods, are exposed to 'geopathic stress'. This phenomenon is said to be a result of natural radiation rising up through the Earth, which is then distorted by electro-magnetic fields created by underground streams, mineral deposits and fault lines. The distortion interacts with our own energy field – or with that of our dogs – to create chronic illness.

I know of several families where persistent illness was evident in both the family members and their pets, and for whom a move of house seemed to bring a new lease of life to all concerned. I am not suggesting moving home whenever chronic disease occurs, but persistent illness that is affecting an entire household for no apparent reason could suggest the possibility of geopathic stress as a factor. A device that can be fitted in the home to neutralize geopathic radiation is now available.

lifestyle

Providing the perfect environment for your dog will be pointless unless he or she also leads a healthy life. Exercise is essential for all dogs, although different types and breeds of dog obviously have different requirements: for instance, a young border collie will need many more walks and runs than an elderly great dane.

hygiene

Thorough grooming is also important. The amount of grooming that is required will depend on the type, length and thickness of a dog's coat, but daily brushing will help to keep even the coat of a short-haired breed in top condition.

You should also develop the habit of examining your dog on a regular basis. Look carefully at his or her eyes, ears and nose for any signs of inflammation or discharge, and check the teeth for discoloration or tartar formation. Take note of any abnormal smells emanating from the ears, skin or breath. Move your hands over the dog's body and feel for any unusual lumps or swellings, and check the skin for signs of fleas or other parasites. If you get to know what your dog looks, smells and feels like, you will notice any abnormality at an early stage and will be able to take prompt and appropriate action. You should also familiarize yourself with the appearance of his or her urine and faeces: any sudden changes in either could be significant and a visit to your vet may be necessary.

A dog's bedding should be frequently laundered, not only for basic hygiene reasons. If an individual suffers from a persistent skin condition, an allergic reaction to the bedding may be the cause, and the bedding may need to be replaced. Your vet can carry out skin tests to determine an allergy of this kind.

nutrition

Take one demanding dog, one overworked, tired owner, one supermarket shelf marked 'pet foods' – and who could resist reaching for a bag of dried food, or for a convenient can? That is, until a problem arises. Take one distressed dog with diarrhoea, one equally distressed owner and one holistic vet, and the advice may well be to resist the 'convenient can' temptation.

commercial dog foods

There is no doubt that many health disorders in dogs can be prevented or cured by paying attention to the diet. So what is in that can or that bag of food that may be less than positive for our dogs?

Water Many canned, or 'moist', foods have a water content of up to 80 per cent ('semi-moist foods contain up to 50 per cent water; 'dry' foods 5–10 per cent water). Apart from the fact that the water itself – if not filtered or pure – could be potentially harmful, a high water content can predispose some dogs to loose bowel movements.

Additives Most canned foods also contain artificial flavouring and colouring. A good food should be tasty enough for a dog to eat without the addition of flavouring and, as dogs do not see colour as we do, any colouring added is for our benefit. Sodium nitrate, for instance, imparts a nice rosy colour to the food, but has been linked to disease in dogs.

BHA and BHT are two preservatives that health experts believe can create liver and kidney problems. Other contaminants, such as hormones and antibiotics, are also sometimes found due to the use of meat from intensively reared livestock. Salt and sugar at unacceptably high levels occasionally occur, especially in 'semi-moist' dog foods.

Labelling Reading the label of a prepared dog food may be confusing. For instance, different brands may have the same level of protein, but not all protein is the same: the protein obtained from meat by-products – including items such as feathers, hair and even leather – are less nutritious than those from 'real' meat. The different types of protein have different biological usefulness to the body, and different digestibility.

For such reasons, it is very difficult to compare like with like in dog foods, or to calculate their actual nutritional value. Manufacturers do not go out of their way to produce sub-standard food for dogs, but ingredients may not always be the healthiest or the best available.

When using proprietary foods, you should therefore look for quality ingredients, with as few by-products, colourings, flavourings and preservatives as possible, and low sugar and salt levels. You may prefer to use dried foods, to which you can add your own water, but there are some good canned foods available. Above all, the food must be palatable. If your dog dislikes it, he or she may well scavenge food from elsewhere and ruin the balanced diet that you are trying to feed.

a vegetarian diet

Is it possible to feed a dog safely on a vegetarian diet? This question is sometimes asked by vegetarian owners who cannot face the idea of preparing meat for their charges. It is quite practicable to feed a dog

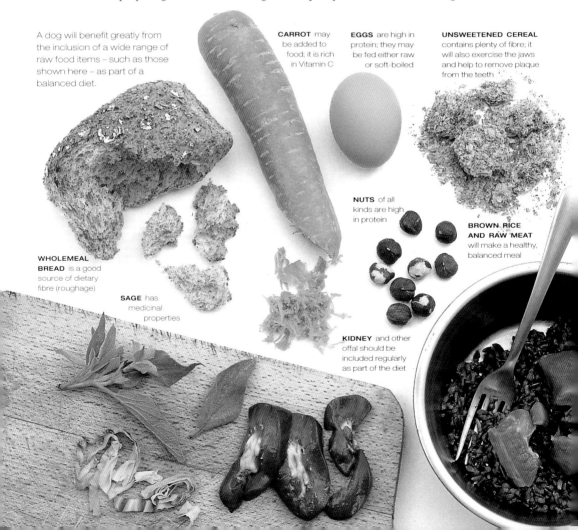

A dog will benefit greatly from the inclusion of a wide range of raw food items – such as those shown here – as part of a balanced diet.

CARROT may be added to food; it is rich in Vitamin C

EGGS are high in protein; they may be fed either raw or soft-boiled

UNSWEETENED CEREAL contains plenty of fibre; it will also exercise the jaws and help to remove plaque from the teeth

NUTS of all kinds are high in protein

BROWN RICE AND RAW MEAT will make a healthy, balanced meal

WHOLEMEAL BREAD is a good source of dietary fibre (roughage)

SAGE has medicinal properties

KIDNEY and other offal should be included regularly as part of the diet

on vegetarian food only, but it has to be said that most dogs really do enjoy meat. Although they are omnivorous rather than truly carnivorous, I suspect that they have stronger leanings towards meat.

However, there are may dogs living happy, healthy vegetarian lives. Some very good commercial vegetarian diets are available, although many contain soya protein which can cause flatulence. It can be rather more difficult to create a home-prepared vegetarian diet that is nutritionally balanced: if you wish to take this option, you should ask your vet for further advice.

a home-made diet

Having looked at why it might be a good idea not to give processed foods, what is the alternative? There is, in my view, no single perfect diet. Variations in size, age and metabolism, and in taste preference, mean that a diet that suits one dog will not necessarily suit another.

CABBAGE should be fed raw in order to preserve its vitamins

It seems sensible, when feeding a natural, home-produced diet, to keep it as close to the food intake of the wild dog as is practicable. The wild dog will kill its prey, and eat it raw, often starting with the internal organs (such as the intestines, liver and heart) and consuming the meat and bones later. The intestines also contain vegetable matter and grains eaten by prey animals. Wild dogs also scavenge for roots, berries and insects. Although a carnivore in structure, the dog is omnivorous by nature, and will consume a large quantity of vegetable matter in a day's hunting.

We do not generally send our dogs out to hunt for food, but a diet similar to that of the wild dog is ideal in principle. If you do not like the idea of feeding raw bones, grains and vegetables, a modified version may be more acceptable and still very healthy. The main priority is to achieve a balanced, nutritious diet, and this should consist of the following items.

Meat This should constitute approximately 40 per cent of the meal. Raw meat is ideal (especially if organically produced), as cooking will denature and destroy some of the nutrients. The exceptions to this rule are raw pork and rabbit, which may contain parasites. If possible, give some of the meat in sizable chunks, as it is good exercise for a dog's jaws to chew at large pieces of meat.

Include fish and chicken or turkey as part of the meat content, as a diet composed mainly of red meat can seem to aggravate hyperactive or even aggressive behaviour in some dogs. Offal – to imitate the consumption of the internal organs in the wild – should also be a part of the meat content. Heart, tripe, kidneys and liver in small amounts are all suitable (raw liver should never be given in large quantities, as an overdosage of Vitamin A could occur). Up to 25 per cent of the meat ration can be given as offal.

Other ingredients The remaining 60 per cent of diet should include vegetables, fruit, pulses, nuts and grains. A variety of foods are suitable, including cooked brown rice, wholemeal bread, chopped nuts, grated raw vegetables such as carrots, unsweetened cereals and fruit. Grains and pulses will be digested better after cooking, simulating the fact that the vegetable matter in the digestive tract of a wild dog's prey will be partially digested.

additional foods

A natural, nutritionally balanced diet should also contain some or all of the following foods, given in the quantities suggested here.

Eggs These are useful as part of a natural, balanced diet. They can be given raw or soft-boiled. One egg per week will be adequate for a small dog; two to three per week for a larger dog.

Live yoghurt This is not only a nutritious food in itself, but the natural bacteria will help the digestive tract to function efficiently. 5 ml (1 tsp) daily is ideal for a small dog; up to 15 ml (3 tsps) for a larger dog.

Milk can be given in small quantities, but it is not a particularly natural food for dogs. In addition, some dogs have difficulty in digesting the lactose in milk, resulting in diarrhoea.

Natural oils Adding 5 ml (1 tsp) of sesame, sunflower or safflower oil to food once or twice weekly will help to balance the diet.

bones

Should dogs be given bones to eat? Every vet who has had to operate to remove a bone obstructing a dog's intestine has mixed views on bones. There is no doubt in my mind that, in principle, bones are good: they are a good source of calcium, help to keep teeth clean, and act as roughage for the digestive tract. Even more importantly, dogs enjoy them! However, there are several very important rules. If you give bones, they must be big, meaty marrow bones, not the type that can splinter and perforate the lining of the intestines. You must also give them raw, as dogs have an innate ability to digest raw bones, but have problems with cooked bones. There is increasing evidence that the best natural diet of all is one composed mainly of raw meaty bones, vegetables and good-quality table scraps. However, if you cannot face the idea of feeding your dog on a bone-based diet, read on.

how much to feed

The age, breed, size, resting metabolic rate and amount of exercise that a dog takes will all affect his or her feeding requirements. A combination of common sense and, if necessary, advice from your vet should indicate the approximate volume of food required. From then onwards, simply watch weight, and energy. If your dog is becoming overweight and is lethargic, cut back on the calories; if his or her weight increases, increase the amount of food. If any weight loss persists, or a weight increase is not controlled by a reduction in food intake, seek veterinary advice.

Obesity is one of the main factors involved in the onset of arthritis, diabetes, liver problems, skin troubles and heart disorders in middle-aged and older dogs, yet no dog is born to be overweight. If obesity is a problem with your dog, your vet will help you to plan and maintain a programme of weight reduction. Treats and titbits are perfectly acceptable – as long as they are wholesome and non-fattening. Most dogs brought up on a piece of apple or carrot as a treat will be just as happy with their titbits as those given 'doggy chocs'.

Remember that growing puppies, working, pregnant and elderly dogs all have different nutritional requirements. The guidelines given here are for an average, adult, healthy dog only. Always consult your vet before implementing dietary changes, especially if your dog has any ongoing health problems, or a past history of recurrent illness.

drinking water

A common concern is whether water should be available at the same time as – or mixed with – food, or given separately. There is some evidence that water drunk with food may reduce the absorption of some minerals (in the wild, dogs usually tend to drink some time apart from eating). My own preference is to keep water constantly available; the dog can then choose when and how much to drink. This water should be changed regularly so that it is always fresh and clean.

supplements

Dietary supplements can be helpful in overcoming any possible deficiencies in a dog's food intake. There are two types: nutritional supplements such as vitamins and minerals, which balance the diet or add 'missing' ingredients; and health supplements, which can enhance the immune system or help to fight infection, but may have no direct nutritional benefit.

nutritional supplements

In theory, if an adult dog is eating a balanced diet of high-quality ingredients, no other supplements should be necessary, but in practice even a home-produced diet may contain ingredients that are lower in vitamins or minerals than is ideal. Certainly, commercial dog foods – even with added vitamins and minerals – may still lose some vitamin content during processing and storage. Young, pregnant, working, ill or old dogs in particular may have special needs for certain supplements. Those that I find have real merit are as follows.

Kelp This is a powder produced from seaweed, and is rich in minerals (especially iodine). It seems to complement vitamin-rich brewer's yeast to provide an optimum multi-vitamin and -mineral combination from natural sources. The mineral content of kelp helps to maintain the efficient functioning of many body processes, including red-blood-cell production, and hormonal and metabolic reactions. Only ¼ tsp per 5 kg (11 lb) body weight need be given daily.

Vitamin C This vitamin is well-known for accelerating the healing of damaged tissue, and for maintaining healthy immune and circulatory systems, and strong bones and joints. It may also help to minimize the risk of cancer. Although dogs produce some natural Vitamin C, a supplement is desirable, especially as this vitamin is not stored in the body. I would recommend 100 mg daily per 5 kg (11 lb) body weight.

Vitamin E This vitamin helps to fight infection and disease, and to cope with the effects of pollution. It is an antioxidant, and aids in preserving the activity of Vitamin A and fatty acids in food. Wheatgerm oil is a good source of Vitamin E, and promotes a good, glossy coat. This vitamin is also available as capsules.

Be sure to use a natural Vitamin E, rather than a synthetic form (look for the term 'd-alpha tocopherol' on the label), as most vitamins from natural sources are better absorbed and seem more active than their synthetic counterparts. Approximately 25 iu (international units) per 5 kg (11 lb) body weight is a suitable daily dose rate.

Cod-liver oil Apart from its invaluable effect in helping to prevent and treat the symptoms of arthritis, and in promoting a healthy skin and coat, the Vitamins A and D in cod-liver oil act in a myriad of ways. Eyesight, tooth formation, nervous tissue and bones and joints are all parts of the body in which Vitamins A and D assist in developing and maintaining normal function. Vitamin A is also an antioxidant and combats the effects of chemicals and pollutants. Halibut-liver oil is another source of Vitamins A and D, and can be much cheaper.

A suitable dose rate of cod-liver oil is one 100 mg capsule per 5 kg (11 lb) body weight daily. This provides about 1000 iu Vitamin A and 100 iu Vitamin D per capsule, depending on the brand used. Cod-liver oil must never be overused, as excessive amounts of Vitamin A can cause damage to bones and joints.

health supplements

The following supplements can be positive adjuncts to a nutritionally balanced and supplemented diet. In addition to those described here, there is an enormous range of other supplements which are claimed to have health-giving properties for dogs, such as ginseng, ginkgo and propolis. Any or all of these may well be beneficial, but I have only included supplements of which I have personal experience.

Chlorella This green alga is rich in vitamins and minerals. It increases energy, promotes red-blood-cell production and assists healing of damaged tissue. It can also help to strengthen the immune system and enhance the destruction of cancer cells. Chlorella is available in tablet form and as a powder. The normal daily dosage rate for a dog is 250 mg per 5 kg (11 lb) body weight. Reports from owners of regular users talk of improved coat condition, fewer digestive upsets and less incidence of disease.

Royal jelly This is a substance secreted by worker bees to feed the growing larvae of the queen bee. A larva fed on royal jelly will itself become a queen, growing larger, living 50 times longer than a normal bee, and laying up to 2000 eggs per day. Luckily, royal jelly does not have quite such a dramatic effect on dogs, but it is a valuable health supplement. It seems to have a stabilizing action on certain metabolic processes in the body – especially those linked to skin and coat condition, energy, appetite and temperament. Royal jelly also has a peculiar capacity to increase energy levels in a dog who is dull and depressed, yet it will calm a nervous, hyperactive individual. It can improve a poor appetite, but will not encourage overeating. In virtually all cases, it will improve skin and coat condition.

Supplements added to a dog's diet can have positive health-giving results.

Fresh royal jelly gives much better results than freeze-dried version. A dose rate of 100 mg daily is recommended.

GARLIC is well-known as 'nature's disinfectant'; it is also available in capsule form

Garlic As well as being a specific herbal remedy for ailments such as chronic respiratory disease, garlic can be given as a general supplement because of its wide-ranging action in the body. Garlic acts as an anti-infective agent, helps to reduce the level of parasites in dogs (both internal and external), and stimulates normal digestive processes.

Ideally, between ⅓ and one fresh clove of garlic should be given daily, depending on the size of the dog. This should be accepted well by most dogs, especially if finely chopped or grated and mixed with food. Alternatively, garlic capsules are available: 2–6 mg of essential garlic oil seems to give the same effect as ⅓ to one clove of fresh garlic. Odourless garlic capsules are also sold in health-food shops, but I find these less successful in keeping parasites such as fleas at bay.

DRIED YEAST is a good source of B-complex and other vitamins and minerals

Dried yeast This is good natural source of B-complex and other vitamins and minerals. Brewer's yeast is the preferred variety. The B group of vitamins has many functions in the body, including that of helping to fight disease. On average, about 2.5 ml (½ tsp) daily per 5 kg (11 lb) body weight is recommended.

administering tablets

Knowing the dosage rate of a tablet is one thing, but giving tablets can be quite another. If your dog dislikes taking them, here are a few tips that are more likely to achieve success at the first attempt, and therefore to cause your dog the minimum of distress and anxiety.

Before giving a tablet, approach your dog calmly and quietly. If possible, ask an assistant to restrain him or her for you; alternatively, position the dog with his or her back against a solid object (such as a wall or a door) so that he or she cannot back away from you, or on a table with a non-slip surface where you can hold on from behind to prevent struggling. Coating a tablet with a little butter or margarine will help it to slip down the throat more easily.

A special syringe known as a 'pill giver' is useful for administering tablets. It also prevents the possibility of contaminating homoeopathic remedies by touching them with the fingers (see page 15).

using a pill giver

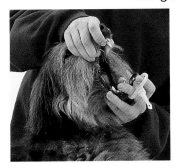

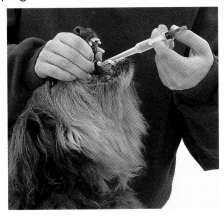

1 Shake the tablet from its container and transfer it to the syringe (be very careful to do this without touching the tablet, to avoid contaminating it and possibly reducing its effectiveness – see page 15). Tilt back the dog's head so that the lower jaw starts to drop, and grasp the upper jaw firmly with your fingers as shown.

2 Pick up the syringe in your free hand, and use it to drop the tablet on to the back of the dog's tongue. (Try to ensure that the tablet falls on the centre of the tongue, as this will make it much more difficult to spit out.) Rub gently down the throat with your fingers to encourage swallowing, then release the dog's head.

common

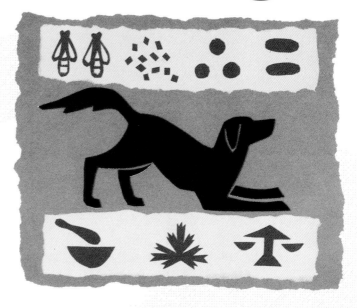

diseases
and conditions

This section covers the main diseases and disorders that dogs may experience, and the natural medicines that can be used to help to relieve the symptoms, or to promote a cure. However, the advice given here is not a substitute for veterinary attention. Any condition that causes your dog to appear seriously unwell, persists for more than a day or two, or has unusual symptoms, needs veterinary advice as soon as possible. Never take risks with your dog's health, and never try to avoid using conventional medicine simply because you prefer natural therapies. Conventional drugs have their drawbacks, but in some cases – for example, when antibiotics are used to treat an acute infection – they can be life-savers.

Although you should never attempt to treat an acute condition solely with natural medicines unless you have been advised to do so by a vet, it is perfectly permissible and indeed a good idea to use them in an emergency while you are waiting for veterinary assistance. Minor problems – small cuts and bruises, mild digestive upsets, itchy skin, and so on – can be safely treated, but if the condition persists you must take your dog to the vet.

This part of the book is designed to help you to understand how natural medicines work, and to make using them easy and effective. It begins with vital instructions on what to do for your dog in emergency situations. This is followed by information on a wide range of the common conditions to affect dogs, which are ordered according to body systems: for example, sprains and strains will be found in the musculo-skeletal system, and vomiting in the digestive system. Each condition has a brief explanation of what it is, how it is caused and what the typical symptoms may be, followed by advice on the natural remedies that will help to treat it.

For information on the dosage and administration of the remedies, refer to the *natural therapies* section on pages 8–37.

emergencies

When a serious accident or other emergency occurs it is all too easy to panic, so a plan of action is invaluable. Natural medicines should be an integral part of this plan, but first aid and the other measures described here may be required initially. Familiarize yourself with the advice given in this section so that, in the event of an emergency, you will know how to care for your dog in the best way possible. Do not give an injured dog anything to eat or drink unless on veterinary advice, in case surgery is required.

emergency action

Keep a clear head and take the following steps in the event of an accident or other emergency.

assess the situation

Check whether the injured dog is conscious, is still breathing and has a heartbeat, by the following means:

• A conscious dog will react to a sudden noise, to pinching of the skin between the toes, or by blinking if a hand is passed in front of his or her eyes.

• To check for breathing, watch the chest closely to see whether it is rising and falling, or hold a feather in front of the dog's nose.

• To feel for a heartbeat, press your fingers firmly against the chest.

prevent further harm

The action needed here should be obvious: for example, if the dog has been electrocuted, turn off the power supply immediately, *before* handling the dog; if the dog has been burned, move him or her away from the heat source; and direct traffic away from an accident site after road injuries, or very carefully move the dog away from danger, using a makeshift stretcher such as a board or blanket.

contact a vet

Carry out any necessary life-saving procedures first (see opposite). Then contact a vet as soon as possible – have your vet's telephone number available at all times – and make transport arrangements.

restrain the dog

Even a normally gentle dog who is in pain may bite, so keep a muzzle available. (In an emergency, use a length of bandage or a scarf looped over the dog's head and tied behind the ears). Until the dog is moved, cover him or her with a blanket or aluminium foil, to prevent heat loss.

first aid

Having taken the appropriate emergency actions, carrying out any necessary first-aid procedures is the next step. The basic techniques outlined below are not difficult to learn, and could save your dog's life.

clear the airway

If the dog is not breathing, or is choking, check for obstructions to the airway. With the dog on his or her side, open the jaws and gently pull the tongue forward. Remove any debris in the nose, mouth or throat.

carry out artificial respiration

If the dog is not breathing but there is a heartbeat, carry out artificial respiration. Close the dog's mouth and, keeping it closed, gently blow into the nostrils until you see the chest rise. Then let the lungs deflate naturally, before beginning the process again. Repeat this procedure 15 times per minute, or until breathing starts spontaneously.

carry out heart massage

If there is no breathing or heartbeat, alternate 15-second spells of artificial respiration with 15-second periods of heart massage. To do this, use the fingers and thumb of one hand to squeeze the chest wall, compressing the chest strongly, then release. Repeat as frequently as possible (at least once, or preferably twice per second). Alternate heart massage with artificial respiration until the heart restarts, and then continue with artificial respiration until breathing restarts.

control bleeding

• If a wound is bleeding uncontrollably, apply pressure at the point of bleeding. Any padding is suitable – sterility is not a priority in an emergency. Apply absorbent padding, overlaid by as many layers of firm bandaging material as necessary, until the bleeding stops.

• If an object – such as a piece of glass – is protruding from the wound, do not try to pull it out as you may cause further damage. Instead, make a ring-shaped pad by twisting a length of material into a doughnut shape, and place this around the wound before gently bandaging the pad in position.

• Only bandage a wound if the bleeding is severe. Contrary to popular belief, you should not apply a tourniquet above the bleeding point: this can obstruct the blood supply to healthy tissue and cause permanent damage. Raising the dog's hindquarters, using a cushion or rolled-up towel, will assist the blood flow to the heart and head.

wounds

Dogs injure themselves in all kinds of ways. I have been called to attend dogs hit by trains, cars, bicycles and most other methods of transport. They get their tails shut in doors, their feet caught in escalators and their ears torn by brambles. I even once had to deal with a dog who had jumped out of a first-storey window. With any injury, carry out first aid as necessary (see page 53), then make use of the valuable assistance of natural medicines.

aromatherapy

Lavender and Terebinth may be massaged in the region of – but not on the site of – a wound.

homoeopathy

Arnica (acute dosage) is the perfect tissue-trauma remedy. This will prevent or minimize bruising, help to stop any bleeding as quickly as possible, and accelerate the healing of damaged and traumatized tissue. Calendula (in the form of lotion or ointment) may be applied directly to an abrasion or laceration using clean cotton wool to promote healing.

wrapping a wound

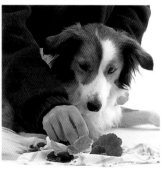

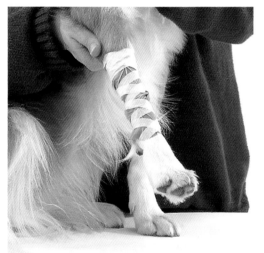

1 Geranium leaves may be wrapped around a wound in order to aid the healing process. For maximum effect, the leaves should be picked just prior to use (or stored for no more than four hours in a refrigerator, to keep them fresh). You will also need a roll of medical adhesive tape and a pair of round-ended scissors.

2 Cut the strips of tape ready for use. Position the leaves over the wound and secure them with tape, taking great care not to apply this too tightly. Replace with fresh leaves daily.

herbal medicine

An infusion of Blackberry may be applied directly to a wound. Another good remedy is to wrap Geranium leaves around the wound or an area of bruising to promote rapid healing (see opposite, below).

Bach flowers

Rescue Remedy, given by mouth in single drops, is always helpful for alleviating shock following an injury of any kind.

minor therapies

biochemical tissue salts

Ferr. phos. (acute dosage) may be administered by mouth, or applied directly to the affected area.

Chinese medicine

Chives are very helpful: the juice of the crushed leaves and roots can be applied to the site of a bruise or laceration to speed healing.

crystals and gems

Pearl (liquid-gem remedy) may be given in single drops by mouth.

bites and stings

Other dogs are the main culprits of bite wounds, although a cornered cat or rat – or even a snake – may bite a dog in self-defence. Bites can become infected, and should be cleaned with a veterinary antiseptic solution before being treated as described below. Insect stings are very common, particularly in the spring and autumn. Puppies have a particular penchant for chasing buzzing insects. If the area around a sting is hot and red, bathe it with cold water, or apply a cold compress (an ice pack or a bag of frozen peas).

aromatherapy

Lavender will be soothing if massaged around a bite or sting, but should not be applied to an open wound.

homoeopathy

Apis mel. is soothing for a sting if the area is swollen and red; Hypericum will relieve a painful bite or sting; and Arnica may be used for a bite that has resulted in an open wound and bruising (all in acute dosage).

herbal medicine

An infusion of Rosemary can be used either for a bite or for a sting.

This should not be applied to an open wound, but used gently to bathe the surrounding area.

Bach flowers

Rescue Remedy, administered as single drops by mouth, will help to calm and quieten a dog who is frightened or distressed.

minor therapies

biochemical tissue salts

Nat. mur. may be applied locally to the site of an insect sting; Ferr. phos. to a bite wound (both remedies to be given in acute dosage).

haemorrhaging

Severe bleeding may be the result of a road-traffic or other accident, a puncture wound or a dog bite. The canine body has an effective blood-clotting mechanism, but, if a major blood vessel is severed, a life-threatening haemorrhage may occur. Immediate first aid should be carried out as necessary (see page 53).

aromatherapy

Lavender may be massaged near – but not directly on – the site of the haemorrhage.

homoeopathy

Arnica (acute dosage) is a superb remedy to help in stopping a serious haemorrhage rapidly. Hamamelis (acute dosage) is useful for the slow seepage of dark, venous blood, rather than the acute 'spurting' of bright-red arterial blood; it is also a good remedy for a haemorrhage inside the earflap (see page 67).

herbal medicine

If the compresses and bandages used to apply pressure at the point of haemorrhage are soaked in an infusion of Meadowsweet and/or Rosemary, the bleeding should cease more quickly.

Bach flowers

Rescue Remedy may be administered in single drops by mouth to counter the shock associated with bleeding.

minor therapies

biochemical tissue salts

Ferr. phos. (acute dosage) may be given by mouth, or powdered tablets may be applied directly to the site of the bleeding.

Chinese medicine

Eggshells – powdered and applied to the bleeding point – will aid clotting; so too will baked, dried chicken (should you have any to hand!).

crystals and gems

Pearl (liquid-gem remedy) may be given as single drops by mouth.

stopping bleeding with Arnica

George and Henry were two labradors – brothers – who loved each other dearly. Except when food was on offer. If they were not kept separated when feeding time came around, fights would inevitably flare up.

I was called to my clinic one evening to find George literally spouting with blood from a bite wound over one eye, with a massive swelling coming up. While I prepared my instruments, assuming that I would have to anaesthetize George, and ligate (tie off) the bleeding vessel, I instructed his owner to give him a dose of Arnica by mouth every two minutes.

By the time I was ready, the bleeding had stopped and the swelling was going down. We reduced the Arnica dosing to 10-minute intervals, and waited for a further 30 minutes. By then there was no swelling, no bleeding and nothing at all to stop George from going home. I gave his owner a phial of Arnica tablets to take with him – ready for the next time.

collapse and shock

A dog in shock may be unconscious or semi-conscious, with pale or bluish gums and shallow breathing. Possible causes could be involvement in a road-traffic accident, electrocution, a diabetic coma, or even heart failure. Heart 'attacks' and coronary heart disease are rare in dogs, but other heart defects will occasionally cause collapse. So too will anaphylactic shock: an acute allergic reaction to stings, drugs or – in rare instances – to food. Give immediate first aid (see page 53), and keep the dog warm until veterinary help arrives.

homoeopathy

Aconite is helpful in all cases of shock, and may be powdered into the mouth of an unconscious patient. Carbo vegetabilis is ideal for a dog who has collapsed but who is still conscious and shows a desire for fresh air. Ver. alb. should be given to a dog who has collapsed and feels very cold to the touch, with bluish gums; it will also help to reduce diarrhoea, a common accompanying symptom. (All three remedies should be given in acute dosage.)

herbal medicine

An infusion of Elder blossom is suitable for a victim recovering from shock. However, this should not be given to an unconscious or semi-conscious patient, as it could be inhaled rather than swallowed.

Bach flowers

Rescue Remedy is ideal for shock and collapse, and should help to promote a rapid recovery. Single drops of the remedy may be applied directly into the mouth of an unconscious dog.

minor therapies

biochemical tissue salts

Nat. sulph. (acute dosage) may be powdered into the mouth of an unconscious dog.

crystals and gems

Pearl (liquid-gem remedy) may be effective: this can be administered as single drops by mouth to a conscious or unconscious dog.

natural remedies alleviate shock

Bruno the dalmation puppy had taken to chasing bees, and one day he finally caught one. He yelped, pawed at his mouth – and within a few seconds collapsed. His breathing slowed, his gums went white, and his owners feared that he was dying.

My instructions over the telephone were to give homoeopathic Aconite (one tablet every two minutes), alternating with Rescue Remedy (one drop every other minute). By the time I arrived Bruno was up and about, although still rather subdued. An examination revealed the bee sting in his lip, but nothing else untoward. Within a few minutes he was back to normal, and had no repercussions – although he has kept a safe distance from bees ever since.

poisoning

Dogs are prone to eating a wide variety of poisonous materials. If you believe that your dog has swallowed a poison your first thought may be to make him or her sick, but if the poison is a strong acid or alkali, or is oil-based, this may be harmful. If you are certain that the poison is not acidic, alkaline or oil-based, induce vomiting by making the dog swallow a piece of washing soda (sodium carbonate), or a concentrated salt solution at a rate of 5 ml (1 tsp) every five minutes for a small dog, 10 ml (2 tsps) for a large dog, until vomiting occurs. If the dog does not vomit within 15 minutes, stop and wait for veterinary help to arrive.

acid, alkali and oil-based poisons

battery acid
bleach
dishwasher detergent
drain cleaner
motor oil
oven cleaner
paint thinners and stripper
paraffin, petrol
polish
toilet cleaner
washing detergent

Administer bicarbonate of soda, egg white or vegetable oil (acid poisons); egg white, vinegar or lemon juice (alkali poisons); and any natural remedies as advised (oil-based poisons).

other poisons

anti-freeze
aspirin and paracetamol
insecticide
mouse, rat and slug bait

Induce vomiting if the poison has been recently swallowed.

aromatherapy

Mint given by massage will hasten recovery from poisoning.

homoeopathy

Aconite is ideal for shock associated with poisoning. Nux vomica is useful following consumption of poisonous plants and Strychnine-based poisons. Ver. alb. may be given where the poisoning results in collapse, a cold body and diarrhoea. (All remedies to be given in acute dosage.)

herbal medicine

An infusion of Hyssop will assist recovery, but should not be given to an unconscious dog. Ipecac. induces vomiting (when appropriate).

Bach flowers

Rescue Remedy administered by mouth will help to overcome shock.

minor therapies

Chinese medicine

Honey may be given at a rate of 5 ml (1 tsp) every 15 minutes for four hours (only to a conscious dog).

burns

Burns are generally caused by heat or boiling liquids, but electrical burns sometimes occur, as do caustic burns resulting from contact with certain chemicals. Do not apply butter or vegetable oil to a burn as – contrary to popular belief – this will not help, but do bathe a burn liberally with cold water before applying a cold compress (an ice pack or a bag of frozen peas).

aromatherapy
Lavender and Rosemary may be massaged around the site of a burn.

homoeopathy
Cantharis (acute dosage) is a good pain-relieving remedy.

Bach flowers
Rescue Remedy will alleviate shock and fright caused by a burn.

minor therapies
biochemical tissue salts
Kali mur. (acute dosage) may be given by mouth, or dissolved in cold water to make a lotion and then applied directly to the burn.
Chinese medicine
Fresh ginger juice, aloe juice and pumpkin pulp are all effective remedies: these should be applied directly to the burn.

heatstroke

Exposure to direct sun, or being left in a car – even on a day that is only 'warm' – can precipitate heatstroke. Very young and old dogs are most at risk, as are overweight individuals and those with long coats. A heatstroke victim should be cooled as rapidly as possible by immersion in cold water (with the head above water), or by hosing for at least one hour or until veterinary help arrives. Place an ice pack or bag of frozen peas on the head to cool the brain. Give plenty of cold water to drink, unless this causes vomiting.

aromatherapy
Mint may be massaged into the skin, especially in the head and neck area.

homoeopathy
Aconite will alleviate shock and early heatstroke. Belladonna is another good remedy (both in acute dosage).

Bach flowers
Rescue Remedy will alleviate shock.

minor therapies
biochemical tissue salts
Nat. mur. and Ferr. phos. (acute dosage) should be given alternately.
Chinese medicine
Radish, bitter gourd (wild cucumber) and wax gourd (winter melon) are ideal. Give 3–4 tsps of any of these foods, well-chopped (however, you should not attempt to do so if the dog is unconscious).

skin

I see more referral cases for skin disorders in dogs than for all other problems put together. The skin is the part of a dog's body with the largest variety of persistent, recurrent problems that are most likely to fail to respond to conventional treatment – I have treated some individuals who have been on fairly continuous medication for skin disease for over a decade. While natural medicines may not resolve all cases of this kind, their success rate is surprisingly high. Skin problems are rarely cured permanently, but natural medicines often achieve long-term remission of the symptoms.

acute eczema

Some of the many causes of this condition (also known as dermatitis) include parasites (see pages 115–16), a bacterial or yeast infection, allergies, injuries (including contact with chemicals) and auto-immune skin diseases. The following remedies are very helpful for 'wet' eczema and infected eczema (pyoderma).

Signs and symptoms Acute inflammation, redness, painful, smelly sores and itching of the skin.

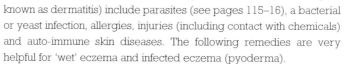

aromatherapy

A combination of Rosemary and Lavender, or of Terebinth, Lavender and Pine, may be massaged into the skin (although not directly into infected, wet or very inflamed areas).

homoeopathy

Hypericum with Calendula tincture may be diluted (three drops per 15 ml [3 tsps] of sterile water) and then applied directly to the skin. The following (all acute dosage) may also provide relief: Apis mel. for allergic reactions and swollen, shiny skin; Cantharis for burning, painful skin eruptions; Hepar sulph. for infected skin (pyoderma); Psorinum for hot, smelly, itchy skin (if the dog prefers to lie in the heat); and Sulphur for hot, itchy skin (if the dog chooses to lie in cool places).

sulphur eases symptoms

Taylor was a well-bred West Highland white terrier, but like many of his breed he was troubled by his skin. Throughout his seven years of life he had been afflicted by itchiness, rashes and hot, uncomfortable skin. However, when I first saw him he had exceeded all previous outbreaks of eczema: his skin was hot to the touch, he could not stop scratching for a second, and it was difficult to say who was more frantic – Taylor or his owners.

A combination of homoeopathic Sulphur by mouth (given in acute dosage) and Aloe vera gel (applied to the worst-affected areas of skin, three times daily) had the acute symptoms under control within two or three days. We are still trying to find a long-term cure for Taylor's tendency to recurrent eczema, but, as with many skin disorders, it takes time and patience to find the most effective remedies.

herbal medicine

A decoction or infusion of Oak bark, or a decoction of Mallow, may be applied as a compress to affected areas. Aloe vera gel, also applied directly, will soothe inflamed and reddened skin. Camomile may be given as an infusion by mouth.

Bach flowers

Crabapple will improve dirty-looking, infected skin, and may also help when the dog is depressed and miserable. Impatiens is beneficial for a nervous, excitable dog whose skin feels hot and is very itchy.

minor therapies

biochemical tissue salts

Ferr. phos. (acute dosage) will help to relieve the symptoms.

Chinese medicine

Spinach, asparagus and crab may be given (1–3 tsps daily, depending on the size of dog).

crystals and gems

Sapphire (liquid-gem remedy) may be given by mouth or added to water.

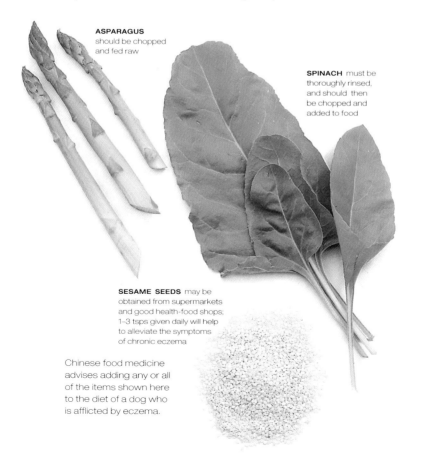

ASPARAGUS should be chopped and fed raw

SPINACH must be thoroughly rinsed, and should then be chopped and added to food

SESAME SEEDS may be obtained from supermarkets and good health-food shops; 1–3 tsps given daily will help to alleviate the symptoms of chronic eczema

Chinese food medicine advises adding any or all of the items shown here to the diet of a dog who is afflicted by eczema.

chronic eczema

The symptoms of this longstanding skin condition often respond well to the natural medicines listed below.

Signs and symptoms Persistent itchiness and soreness, often with hair loss. The skin usually remains dry and flaky, but in some cases may be greasy (seborrhoea).

aromatherapy

A combination of Cedar, Thyme and Lavender, or of Rosemary and Lavender, used for massage, will reduce inflammation.

homoeopathy

The following remedies may all be given in chronic dosage: Acid. nit. for inflammation where the skin meets mucous membranes (such as at the lips and anus); Ant. crud. for scabs on the skin, with a sticky secretion beneath; Arsen. alb. for dry, flaky skin (if the dog prefers the heat); Lycopodium for thickened skin with hair loss; Urtica for itchy, 'nettle-rash' symptoms; Nat. mur. for dry, itchy skin, especially at the bends of the limbs; and Pulex for flea allergies.

herbal medicine

Evening primrose oil is beneficial when combined with cod-liver oil. Nettle, Dandelion and Meadowsweet may be given as infusions. Juniper, Beech, Birch and Pine may be used as herbal tar on the skin (only with the guidance of a herbalist).

Bach flowers

Crabapple will cleanse the skin.

minor therapies

biochemical tissue salts

Kali sulph. is beneficial for greasy skin; Nat. mur. for very dry skin (both in chronic dosage).

Chinese medicine

1–3 tsps of sesame seeds (depending on the dog's size) may be given daily.

alopecia

There are no instant cures for hair loss, although natural remedies can help to promote hair growth on thinning or bald patches. Alopecia may result from a hormonal imbalance, a poor diet, injury, allergies, immune-system disease, infections, parasites or ageing.

Signs and symptoms Hair loss may be generalized, or in patches. If the balding is bilaterally symmetrical (the same on either side), the cause is likely to be hormonal.

aromatherapy

Rosemary may be used for massage, or given via a diffuser. Alternatively, any of the following combinations –

Lavender with Calamus, with Terebinth and Pine, or with Thyme and Cedar – are suitable, and should be massaged into hairless areas.

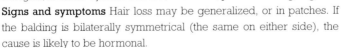

homoeopathy

The following may be used (all in chronic dosage): Sepia alternating with Pulsatilla (for female hormonal hair loss); Lycopodium for the prematurely grey, ageing and balding dog; and Arsen. alb. for loss of coat with itchiness and dandruff. Thallium is a good general homoeopathic hair restorer.

herbal medicine

Apple-cider vinegar may be added to drinking water at the rate of 5 ml (1 tsp) per 600 ml (1 pt). Dandelion makes a good infusion for alopecia. Burdock-root oil may be beneficial when massaged directly into the skin, especially if the skin is particularly dry and scurfy (scaling). Nettle with Birch and Burdock can also be used for massage.

minor therapies

biochemical tissue salts

Kali sulph. is helpful for bald areas with moist, slightly sticky skin; Nat. mur. is suitable for bald areas with dry, scurfy skin; and Silica for balding areas that have a dull, non-glossy appearance.

crystals and gems

Sapphire (liquid-gem remedy) may be given by mouth or added to water.

supplements

Seaweed and kelp powder are rich sources of minerals; either of these may be added to food daily.

anal-gland disorders

The anal glands are two scent glands located on either side of the anal ring. Many dogs are prone to suffering from blocked glands, which can lead to irritation and infection. The causes are unknown, although too little fibre (roughage) in the diet may predispose blockages. Blocked anal glands will need to be emptied by a vet.

Signs and symptoms Itchiness around the anus is typical: an affected dog may shuffle his or her bottom along the ground, or may suddenly look around as though feeling a shooting pain.

homoeopathy

Hepar sulph. (acute dosage) may be given if the glands are infected, and Silicea (chronic dosage) for blockages that occur repeatedly.

herbal medicine

Garlic (⅓ to one chopped clove) should be added to food daily.

minor therapies

biochemical tissue salts

Calc. phos. given alternately with Nat. mur. (both in acute dosage) will help to relieve the symptoms in a case of acute inflammation and blockage. Silica (chronic dosage) is suitable for a chronic recurrent blockage of the anal glands.

warts

Warts are usually harmless, but may become infected or bleed if damaged. They may be caused by a viral infection, or simply occur as part of the ageing process. Some dogs develop large 'crops' of warts.
Signs and symptoms Warts may range in shape from 'cauliflower-like' to sessile (flat).

homoeopathy

Thuja tincture should be applied as one drop on each wart daily. Causticum (chronic dosage) will be beneficial for an old, stiff, warty dog.

herbal medicine

Greater-celandine juice, or slices of Garlic or Banana skin, may be applied to a wart (see below). Milk thistle may be given as an infusion.

minor therapies

biochemical tissue salts

Kali mur. may be used alternately with Nat. mur. (both to be given in chronic dosage).

Chinese medicine

Peanuts and brown sugar, ground together, make a good infusion.

crystals and gems

Coral (liquid-gem remedy) may be given by mouth or added to water.

covering a wart

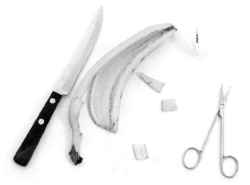

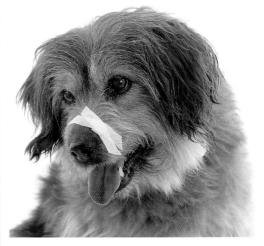

1 Banana skin is a very good remedy for eliminating warts, and often produces rapid results. Simply cut a square of freshly peeled Banana skin, large enough to cover the surface of the wart and the area surrounding it. Cut a piece of medical adhesive tape to the length required, and put this to one side ready for use.

2 Place the Banana skin over the wart, and secure it with tape (taking great care not to apply this too tightly if around a limb). Replace with fresh Banana skin daily.

abscess

An abscess may actually be under the skin rather than within it, but it is at the skin's surface that it will be visible. An abscess may develop due to bacterial infection of a bite or wound, or following the penetration of a foreign body. It may be brought to a 'head' and encouraged to discharge the pus within it by applying a proprietary herbal drawing ointment or warm salty water.

Signs and symptoms An abscess is obvious as a painful swelling, which may discharge pus.

aromatherapy
Lavender and St John's wort massaged around the abscess site will have a soothing effect.

homoeopathy
Apis mel. is a good remedy for a hot, red, shiny abscess; Graphites for interdigital cysts, caused by infection between the toes; Hepar sulph. for an 'active', discharging abscess; and Lachesis for a painful, purplish abscess (all in acute dosage). Silicea (chronic dosage) should help a longstanding abscess to heal.

herbal medicine
Garlic and Echinacea will hasten the healing process.

Bach flowers
Rock rose is soothing for a very painful abscess.

minor therapies
biochemical tissue salts
Ferr. phos. may be given in the early, acute stage; and Silica while the abscess is discharging (both in acute dosage). Calc. phos. (chronic dosage) will help subsequent healing.

Chinese medicine
Castor beans – ground and applied to the abscess – will promote healing (these must not be given by mouth).

two remedies cure abscess

Ferdinand was a bull terrier of great strength, but of equal gentleness. He had no aggression in him, and, when attacked and bitten by a rampaging Yorkshire terrier, simply walked away. However, the bite wound did not heal well, and some days later Ferdinand was brought to my surgery with a massive swelling where the bite had been.

'I think' I said, as I pulled the scab from the top of the swelling, 'this could be an abscess.' As the scab came off, a jet of pus gushed out over the table. Ferdinand turned not a hair, but his owner promptly fainted. I cleaned up the wound, prescribed the homoeopathic remedy Hepar sulph. (to be given in acute dosage) and advised massaging lavender essential oil around the wound daily.

Ferdinand was the best of patients, took his tablets, and seemed to enjoy his daily massage. He made a rapid recovery from the abscess, and within a week healing was complete. His owner, however, was still the less-than-proud possessor of a large bump on the forehead.

ears and eyes

Dogs may begin to lose their acute sense of hearing or to suffer from failing eyesight as part of the ageing process, but most cope well with this gradual loss, relying instead increasingly on their powerful sense of smell. Ears and eyes are complicated organs, and any disease should be treated as soon as possible.

In younger dogs, ear problems can occur in three areas: the ear flap, the ear canal, and the middle and inner ear. Individuals of breeds with heavy, hanging ear flaps often suffer particularly from problems due to lack of ventilation in the ear canal. A dog's eyes can become injured or be affected by a range of conditions. Some of the most common disorders of the ears and eyes are included here.

otitis externa

A dog's ear canal is long, narrow and turns inwards towards the ear drum, resulting in poor ventilation. Breeds with hanging ear flaps (such as spaniels) or hairy ears (such as poodles) are particularly prone to hot, sticky ear canals that become inflamed, in a condition known as otitis externa. This may be due to the presence of ear mites (see page 116); to a foreign body such as a grass awn, polyp or tumour; or to a bacterial, fungal or yeast infection.

Signs and symptoms Head-shaking and scratching; discharge and odour at the ear hole.

aromatherapy

Clove and Thyme may be massaged into the skin near the ears to help to soothe inflammation. A good general cleansing agent may be made from 5 ml (1 tsp) of warm Olive oil with a few drops of Lemon juice: this may be used to clean the outer part of the ear. A few drops should be allowed to drain into the ear canal, and the base of the ear massaged. This will soothe the ear, and encourage any excess wax or discharge to come out. Do not attempt to clean inside the ear canal, and never use cotton buds: the tissues are very delicate and are easily damaged.

resolving otitis externa

Suki, like many cocker spaniels, was afflicted by recurrent otitis externa. As soon as summer began, she would start to scratch and shake her ears, they would become red and hot, and an unpleasant aroma would emanate, variously described by her owners as resembling mouldy cheese, unwashed socks and dry rot. Conventional drugs produced only a short-term improvement. I prescribed homoeopathic Psorinum (chronic dosage), which suits a hot, smelly, intensely itchy ear. Suki responded well and, although there was a slight recurrence of the condition the next summer, a few days on Psorinum soon solved the problem. Since then, Suki's ears have remained itch- and smell-free.

homoeopathy

Hypericum with Calendula lotion is a good homoeopathic cleansing agent. For internal use, the following may help (acute dosage in a severe case, chronic dosage in a longstanding one): Graphites for a sticky, smelly discharge; Hepar sulph. when there is an infected, purulent discharge; and Psorinum for a hot, itchy ear (if the dog prefers to be warm), or Sulphur (if the dog prefers to be cool).

herbal medicine

A good herbal cleansing agent comprises three parts Rosemary infusion mixed with one part Witch-hazel lotion. An effective cleansing remedy when ear mites are present (see page 116) is made of equal parts of Thyme, Rosemary and Rue infusions, mixed 50:50 with Olive oil. An infusion of Thyme will soothe inflammation in the ear canal, and so help to reduce scratching and head-shaking attempts to relieve irritation.

minor therapies

biochemical tissue salts

The following are all helpful (acute dosage should be given in a severe case, chronic dosage if the problem is longstanding): Calc. sulph. for a profuse discharge containing blood; Ferr. phos. for an ear that is painful and hot to the touch; or Kali sulph. for yellow, catarrhal discharge.

crystals and gems

Sapphire (liquid-gem remedy) may be given by mouth or added to water.

haematoma

This is a haemorrhage that occurs within the ear flap, causing it to swell. Causes include physical trauma (for example, from banging the ear against a hard object, or trapping it in a door), and parasites or infection in the ear canal. Surgery to drain the haematoma followed by suturing (stitching) of the ear flap to prevent further haemorrhaging is usually advised, although this can often be avoided by the use of natural medicines.

Signs and symptoms Violent head-shaking or head-rubbing, and a swollen ear flap.

homoeopathy

Arnica (to be administered in acute dosage) for three days, followed by Hamamelis (given in chronic dosage) for two weeks, may help to reduce the swelling of the ear flap. (Arnica is an excellent remedy that is also used to reduce bruising following injury.)

herbal medicine

Witch-hazel lotion may be applied directly to the ear flap.

minor therapies

biochemical tissue salts

Ferr. phos. (acute dosage) will help to relieve the symptoms.

otitis media and otitis interna

Most middle- and inner-ear problems are caused by an inward spread of otitis externa (see pages 66–7). Infection can also travel from the throat via the Eustachian tube, which connects the throat to the ear. The causes of otitis media and interna include bacterial, fungal or yeast infection, and (occasionally) tumours.

Signs and symptoms Head-shaking and ear-scratching; a severely affected dog may walk in circles or even fall over, as the condition can affect the sense of balance.

aromatherapy

Rosemary and Thyme essential oils may be used for gentle massage around the base of the ear.

homoeopathy

Hepar sulph. (acute dosage) is an ideal remedy for symptoms that have developed only recently; Merc. cor. (chronic dosage) should be given for a longer-term problem.

Bach flowers

Scleranthus will be helpful if the dog's balance is affected.

minor therapies

biochemical tissue salts

Kali mur. (acute dosage) will alleviate the catarrh that forms in the ear.

crystals and gems

Sapphire (liquid-gem remedy) may be given by mouth or added to water.

conjunctivitis

Conjunctivitis is an inflammation of the pink mucous membrane surrounding the 'white' of the eye. It is a common problem, and may be caused by a viral or bacterial infection, a foreign body, an allergic reaction, entropion (see page 71) or physical trauma.

Signs and symptoms Red, sore-looking eyes with accompanying discharge. The dog may paw at the eyes or rub his or her face along the ground in an attempt to relieve irritation.

homoeopathy

The following may be used: Apis mel. for sore eyes with swollen eyelids and/or swollen conjunctiva; Arsen. alb. for watery, inflamed eyes with a thin but acrid discharge; Kali bich. for a thick, green, stringy discharge; and Pulsatilla for a bland, creamy, catarrhal discharge.

herbal medicine

Greater-celandine or Dock infusion may be used to bathe the eyes three times daily. A fresh infusion should be made each day, and kept cool and covered when not in use. Eyebright – or Goldenseal infusion or diluted tincture – can be used in the same way, or given orally.

minor therapies
biochemical tissue salts
The following will be helpful (all in acute dosage): Ferr. phos. when no discharge is present; Kali mur. for a white discharge; Nat. phos. for a sticky yellow discharge; and Silica where styes (eyelid swellings) are present.
Chinese medicine
Cucumber juice – freshly pressed on each occasion – may be applied directly to the eyes: three drops should be administered to each eye (see below), three times daily. An alternative Chinese food remedy is to add 1–3 tsps (depending on the size of the dog) of diced water chestnut to food twice daily.
crystals and gems
Pearl (liquid-gem remedy) may be helpful: single drops should be given by mouth.

administering eye drops

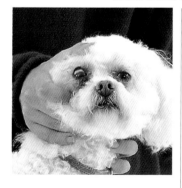

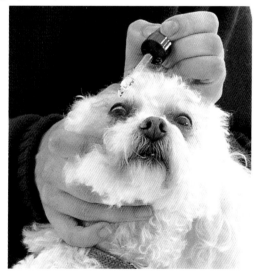

1 Small bottles with droppers in the lids are available from pharmacies. If you wish to re-use a bottle, be sure to clean it very thoroughly with hot water, and then leave it to air-dry before use. Giving eye drops will be easier if you have the help of an assistant to restrain the dog properly; alternatively, position the dog against a solid surface so that he or she is not able to back away from you. Draw up the medicine into the dropper. Use the fingers of one hand to hold the eyelids of one eye open.

2 Taking great care not to hold the dropper too close to the eye in case the dog were to move suddenly, carefully administer the drop or drops. Release the eyelids and allow the dog to blink several times: this will help to disperse the liquid over the surface of the eyeball.

corneal ulceration

The cornea is the central, transparent area of the eye. It is very delicate – even tiny scratches may ulcerate rapidly – and has no direct blood supply, so it heals slowly. An ulcer may be caused by injury, infection, a foreign body, entropion (see opposite), or due to a deficiency in tear production.

Signs and symptoms The eye will be red, sore and discharging. The dog may rub his or her face along the ground, and be photophobic (avoid bright light).

clearing an eye ulcer

Punch was a Lhasa apso with a deep ulcer on the cornea of one eye that was not responding to conventional treatment. When I saw him, the eye was painful and inflamed. I recommended homoeopathic Argent. nit. (acute dosage) for three days, then Eyebright tincture (three drops to be diluted in 10 ml [2 tsps] of sterile water: one drop in the eye three times daily).

After three days the ulcer was starting to heal. The Argent. nit. was reduced to chronic dosage, and the drops given twice daily. The Eyebright was then continued alone (one drop daily) for 10 days until the eye was clear.

homoeopathy

The following remedies will be helpful: Argent. nit. (acute dosage) for a painful eye, with redness and obvious soreness; Merc. cor. for pain and photophobia (the dog may also be thirsty); and Silicea (chronic dosage), for discomfort caused by the scarring of an old ulcer.

herbal medicine

An infusion of Greater celandine may be applied directly to the eye. A diluted tincture or infusion of Eyebright or Goldenseal may also be used in this way, or given orally.

kerato conjunctivitis sicca

More commonly known as 'dry eye', this deficiency in tear production causes the surface of the eye to dry out. West Highland white terriers are often affected. Causes include immune-system deficiencies, eye injury and some drugs (especially salazopyrin, used to treat colitis). Bathing with cold tea three times daily will soothe and cleanse the eye. Cod-liver oil is a good lubricant, and aids healing: three drops should be applied to each eye three times daily.

Signs and symptoms A thick, sticky discharge from reddened, sore eyes, and a dry nose.

homoeopathy

Zinc. met. and Silicea (both given in chronic dosage) will help to relieve the discomfort of this condition.

cataract

This is an opacity of the lens of the eye. For light to be able to travel through the lens it must obviously be transparent, so any opacity will cause defective vision and, if the cataract progresses, blindness. A cataract or cataracts can be a congenital problem (ie present from birth), or may develop as part of ageing. Poisoning, diabetes mellitus (see pages 80–1) and infection can also cause cataracts.

Dog owners are, naturally, concerned about a pet becoming blind but, if cataracts develop slowly, most dogs adjust very well to a gradual loss of sight. It is their sense of smell that is much more important.

Signs and symptoms Obvious visual difficulties, and a blue or white opacity of the lens.

homoeopathy
Cineraria eye lotion should be applied twice daily. The following are also helpful: Calc. carb. for an old, overweight dog; Conium mac. for an old, weak dog, especially with weak hindquarters; and Phosphorus for a thin, older dog.

herbal medicine
An infusion of Greater celandine may be given.

minor therapies
biochemical tissue salts
Nat. mur. is beneficial for recent cataracts, and Silica for established cataracts (each to be administered in chronic dosage).

supplements
Supplementation of the diet with Vitamin E (100–300 iu to be given daily, depending on the size of the dog) and Selenium (25–50 mg daily) will be beneficial.

entropion

This is usually a congenital condition, in which one or more eyelids are curled inwards. This causes the eyelids or eyelashes to rub on the eye, predisposing it to conjunctivitis or corneal ulceration. (Other similar conditions are ectropion, where the eyelid turns out too much, often causing conjunctivitis; and distichiasis, in which extra, inward-growing eyelashes rub on the eye and predispose it to conjunctivitis or corneal ulceration). Surgery is often necessary, but entropion can be improved by the following natural therapies.

Signs and symptoms See conjunctivitis (pages 68–9) and corneal ulceration (see opposite, above).

homoeopathy
Borax (chronic dosage) encourages the eyelids to uncurl, reducing inflammation.

herbal medicine
Rosemary may be administered in the form of an infusion.

glaucoma

Glaucoma is an increase of pressure inside the eyeball. The eye is filled with a fluid that is constantly secreted and drained, but, if anything disturbs this balance, pressure builds up, bringing a rapid risk of permanent damage and blindness. The condition may be caused by congenital abnormalities in drainage, or by infection, inflammation or a tumour.

Signs and symptoms The affected eye will be extremely painful and may be swollen.

homoeopathy
Belladonna or Phosphorus (both remedies to be administered in acute dosage) will reduce inflammation.

uveitis

This is an inflammation of tissues inside the eye – in particular, the iris (the coloured part of the eye). It can be a very painful condition. Possible causes of uveitis are bacterial or viral infection, injury, immune-system abnormalities and tumours in the eye.

Signs and symptoms Obvious pain, photophobia, eye discharge and visible cloudiness in the eye.

homoeopathy
The following may be helpful (all in acute dosage): Phosphorus, if there is internal bleeding in the eyeball; Rhus tox. where there is severe irritation and discomfort; and Symphytum, if the uveitis is the result of an injury to the eye.

epiphora

This condition involves an overflow of tears. It is often the result of conjunctivitis (see pages 68–9) or corneal ulceration (see page 70), although some dogs' eyes permanently water. White dogs are particularly prone to epiphora. Where no other eye disease is present, the usual cause is deficient drainage through the tear duct.

Signs and symptoms Dark tear staining on the dog's face, running from the inner corners of the eyes down the muzzle.

homoeopathy
Allium cepa (acute dosage) will help.

herbal medicine
A diluted tincture or infusion of Eyebright may be used to bathe the eyes twice daily (a fresh solution should be made up each day).

minor therapies
biochemical tissue salts
Nat. mur. (chronic dosage) will help.

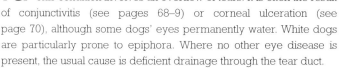

respiratory system

In the winter months, humans are prone to coughs, colds, influenza, bronchitis and various other conditions. Other animals, such as cats, are also particularly prone to these types of problems. Dogs are better adapted to cold climates, and are therefore less prone to respiratory disease: in fact, colds and influenza are virtually unknown in the dog world. However, the following problems of the respiratory tract do arise, especially in situations where many dogs are kept together (such as at boarding kennels).

coughing

Persistent coughing is the most common symptom of respiratory disease, and is particularly irritating for dog and owner alike. It can be caused by numerous factors, including viral infection (especially 'kennel cough' – see page 118), a foreign body in the airway, allergies or physical irritants (such as smoke), lung congestion, tumours or airway parasites (lungworms).

Signs and symptoms The frequent bouts of coughing may be productive (accompanied by mucus) or non-productive (dry).

aromatherapy
Eucalyptus, Hyssop, Myrrh, Pine, Teatree, Terebinth and Thyme will all be effective, and may be used for massage or given via a diffuser.

homoeopathy
The following will all help: Arsen. alb. for harsh coughing that worsens at night; Bryonia for dry coughing that worsens in the morning; Ipecac. syrup for spasmodic coughing, with vomiting; Spongia for coughing linked with a heart problem; Rumex crispus for coughing that improves at night; and Drosera for a sensitive larynx.

herbal medicine
Garlic, Sage, Thyme, Liquorice, Ribwort plantain and Coltsfoot will all be beneficial. Mullein is good for coughing that is worse at night.

minor therapies
biochemical tissue salts
Ferr. phos. (acute dosage) should be given for an acute, dry, hard cough. The following will also help (all in chronic dosage): Calc. sulph. for a loose, rattling cough; Kali mur. for coughing with white mucus; Kali sulph. for yellow mucus; Mag. phos. for spasmodic, persistent coughing ('kennel cough'); and Silica for coughing that is accompanied by a profuse, yellow-green mucus.

Chinese medicine
Ginger, spearmint, grapes and kumquats should be given in small amounts (1 tsp added to a dog's food daily). Other recommended remedies are lemon for coughing accompanied by excessive mucus; strawberries for a dry cough; and pumpkin for bronchial asthma.

sinusitis and nasal discharge

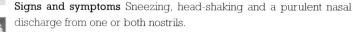

The upper respiratory tract is less often a site for disease in dogs than in humans or even in cats, but, when it does occur, sinusitis is just as annoying a problem. The cause may be infection (bacterial or fungal), or the presence of a foreign body (such as a grass awn) or tumours.

Signs and symptoms Sneezing, head-shaking and a purulent nasal discharge from one or both nostrils.

aromatherapy

Eucalyptus, Hyssop, Myrrh, Pine, Teatree, Terebinth and Thyme may all be given by diffusion or massage.

homoeopathy

The following will be helpful (all in chronic dosage): Kali bich. for a yellow, tough, stringy discharge; Pulsatilla for a bland, catarrhal, profuse discharge; and Silicea for chronic, intractable sinusitis.

herbal medicine

Goldenseal, Garlic and Liquorice will all help to relieve the symptoms.

minor therapies

biochemical tissue salts
The following will be beneficial: Ferr. phos. (acute dosage) for severe sinusitis; Kali mur. (chronic dosage) for catarrhal, white mucus; Kali sulph. (chronic dosage) for a yellow, thick mucus; and Nat. mur. (chronic dosage) for a watery, thin discharge.

Chinese medicine
Cornsilk or onion leaf may be given (1–3 tsps daily, depending on the size of the dog).

crystals and gems
Pearl (liquid-gem remedy) may be given by mouth or added to water.

pneumonia

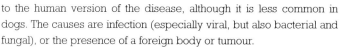

Pneumonia is a serious condition. It has similar symptoms to the human version of the disease, although it is less common in dogs. The causes are infection (especially viral, but also bacterial and fungal), or the presence of a foreign body or tumour.

Signs and symptoms Acute and persistent coughing, rapid breathing, a high fever and chest pain.

aromatherapy

Eucalyptus, Hyssop, Myrrh, Pine, Teatree, Terebinth and Thyme are all soothing remedies that will help to relieve the symptoms. Any or all of these may be used for gentle massage or administered via a diffuser.

homoeopathy

Aconite should be given at the first signs, and Belladonna at the height of fever (both in acute dosage). Bryonia should be given if the dog is unwilling to move; Phosphorus if the condition is painful, with coughed-up blood;

and Sulphur where there is fever and coughed-up yellow mucus.

herbal medicine
Garlic and Nasturtium have a natural anti-infective action.

minor therapies
biochemical tissue salts
Ferr. phos. (acute dosage) is suitable for acute pneumonia; Kali mur. (acute dosage) for pneumonia with a thick mucus and congested lungs; and Silica (chronic dosage) for persistent pneumonia and scarred lungs.
Chinese medicine
Saffron, grapefruit peel, tangerine and beetroot may all be given in small amounts (1–3 tsps daily) while the pneumonia is acute.

using combined remedies
Genevieve was an Afghan hound who had developed 'kennel cough' following a dog show, which progressed into acute pneumonia.

Antiobiotics were already being given, to little effect. I began a programme of twice-daily massage with Eucalyptus and Thyme (which Genevieve adored), homoeopathic Belladonna tablets (acute dosage) which she tolerated, and beetroot juice (Chinese food cure: 10 ml [2 tsps] daily) which she hated. Within three days she was up and about, still coughing a little but already almost back to her old self.

epistaxis

Epistaxis – otherwise known as a nose bleed – is alarming when in full flow, but can often be arrested rapidly with natural medicines. It is frequently caused by injury, or by infection. It may also result from tumours or a foreign body in the nasal passage.
Signs and symptoms The bleeding may come from one or both of the dog's nostrils.

homoeopathy
Arnica (acute dosage) may be given at the start of bleeding, especially if caused by injury. Also beneficial (all in acute dosage) are Ipecac. for bright-red blood, with vomiting; Phosphorus for persistent bleeding; and Melilotus for profuse bleeding.

minor therapies
biochemical tissue salts
Ferr. phos. is a good remedy for epistaxis. This may be administered either by mouth (acute dosage), or the tablets may be crushed and applied directly to the nostrils.
Chinese medicine
Water chestnuts, chives or vinegar may be added to food frequently in small amounts (not more than 5 ml [1 tsp] of vinegar, twice daily, should be given), while the tendency to bleeding persists.
crystals and gems
Pearl (liquid-gem remedy) may be given as single drops by mouth.

cardiovascular system

The diseases in this section cover the heart, and the circulatory system of blood and lymph. Dogs, on the whole, have a healthier lifestyle than humans, so these problems are less commonly seen by vets than by doctors. When they do occur, natural medicines can be very effective at alleviating the symptoms.

heart disease

Dogs are sometimes born with heart defects, and may also experience problems with the control mechanisms of the heart. The most common problem is congestive heart failure. This is caused by a malfunctioning heart valve, infection, or congenital abnormalities, and means that the heart cannot pump enough blood to body tissues. The following medicines are all compatible with any prescribed drugs; it is also wise to reduce salt intake, to encourage weight loss in obese patients, and to promote gentle exercise.

Signs and symptoms Breathlessness, coughing, lethargy (resulting in an unwillingness to exercise), oedema (see opposite), weight loss and liver disease (see page 100).

aromatherapy
Mint given by massage will help heart and circulatory problems.

homoeopathy
The following are beneficial for heart disease (all given in chronic dosage): Crataegus and Digitalis for a weak heart and poor circulation; Spongia tosta and Rumex crispus for any associated coughing; Cactus grand. for pain; Lycopus if the heartbeat is rapid; and Adonis and Strophanthus for valve problems. Laurocerasus is beneficial where the lungs are congested and there is cyanosis (poor oxygenation of the blood); the tincture may also be given (one drop every 15 minutes for up to two hours) where there is a danger of cyanosis.

herbal medicine
Capsicum, Rosemary and Convallaria are all suitable for heart disease: infusions of one or more of these remedies will encourage the removal of excess fluid and more efficient heart function.

minor therapies
biochemical tissue salts
Calc. fluor. (chronic dosage) will improve the strength of the heart muscle; Kali phos. (chronic dosage) stabilizes electric abnormalities.
Chinese medicine
Sweetcorn or wholewheat (1–3 tsps, depending on the size of dog) should be added to food daily.
crystals and gems
Ruby (liquid-gem remedy) may be given by mouth or added to water.

congestion

Many problems in the heart and circulatory system cause a severe build-up of fluid. This congestion, or oedema, may be evident in the form of swollen feet or legs, or as fluid on the lungs or in the abdomen (known as ascites, or dropsy). A failing heart is a common cause of congestion, as the heart is unable to maintain the circulation of blood and excess fluid begins to pool in the tissues. Liver disease (see page 100) and the presence of tumours can also contribute to this type of congestion.

Signs and symptoms Swollen, puffy limbs in particular, or swelling occurring in any part of the body; an enlarged, tense abdomen; weight loss and a general lack of energy and enthusiasm.

aromatherapy

Lemon, Birch, Sandalwood and Juniper essential oils may all be used for gentle massage, and will help to relieve congestion.

homoeopathy

The following are beneficial (all to be administered in chronic dosage): Apis mel. for oedema where the skin shows a visible depression after being pressed, and where the dog is not particularly thirsty; Acetic acid and Eel serum for congestion, especially ascites (fluid on the lungs or in the abdomen), where the dog appears to be fairly thirsty; and Adonis and Digitalis for congestion with major heart disease.

herbal medicine

Bearberry, Dandelion, Dill seed, Ground elder, Hawthorn, Juniper berry, Parsley and Sloe berry, given by infusion, are all ideal for congested circulation (all can be helpful, but no more than two of these remedies are necessary at the same time).

minor therapies

biochemical tissue salts

Calc. sulph. and Nat. sulph. are useful remedies (both to be administered in chronic dosage); the latter will be especially useful where liver disease has contributed to the oedema.

Chinese medicine

Plums (dried), broad-bean pods and mung beans may be given (amounts depend on dog's size): one to two plums on alternate days; one to three broad-bean pods daily; and 1–3 tsps of sprouted mung beans daily.

crystals and gems

Pearl (liquid-gem remedy) may be given by mouth, or added to water.

supplements

If diuretics (drugs to eliminate the excess fluid from the body) are being administered to the dog, a Potassium supplement may also be advisable. This is because the use of diuretics causes an excessive loss of Potassium with the fluid (your vet will give you further advice about whether supplementation with Potassium is advisable).

anaemia

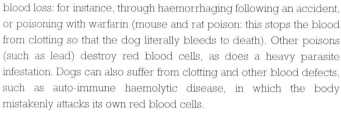

Anaemia is a lack of red blood cells in the body. It results from blood loss: for instance, through haemorrhaging following an accident, or poisoning with warfarin (mouse and rat poison: this stops the blood from clotting so that the dog literally bleeds to death). Other poisons (such as lead) destroy red blood cells, as does a heavy parasite infestation. Dogs can also suffer from clotting and other blood defects, such as auto-immune haemolytic disease, in which the body mistakenly attacks its own red blood cells.

Signs and symptoms Pale lips and gums, and general weakness.

aromatherapy

Marjoram given by massage will assist in rejuvenating a weak, anaemic dog.

conventional and natural cures

Major Tom was a mongrel with an uncertain ancestry: there seemed to be at least a dozen different breeds among his forebears. Despite the general rule that mongrels are more healthy than their pedigree counterparts, Tom was afflicted by an immune-system disease that damaged his red blood cells and caused anaemia, leaving him slow and lethargic.

As well as conventional treatment, I added the following: China officinalis (homoeopathic remedy for debility: chronic dosage); Nettles and Parsley added to food (herbal remedies for anaemia), Hornbeam (Bach flower remedy for strength: one drop daily); Ferr. phos. (tissue salt, to enhance red-blood-cell production: chronic dosage); and mung beans (Chinese food remedy: 1 tsp daily).

Results were gradual, but over six months Tom's red-blood-cell count rose significantly. From then on, he was also given extra liver, kelp, Brewer's yeast and royal jelly. After a further six months the count was almost normal, with the conventional drugs also reduced.

homoeopathy

The following should all be given in chronic dosage: China officinalis for debility; Crotalus horridus for warfarin poisoning; Ferrum met. where poor nutrition is a factor; Cuprum met. where insufficient red blood cells are produced; Lachesis if clotting disorders are causing dark haemorrhages; Lycopodium for excessive destruction of red blood cells (for example, in auto-immune haemolytic disease); Phosphorus where persistent bleeding of bright red blood is contributing to the anaemia; Secale for haemorrhages under the skin; and Acid. phos. to improve weakness, especially in a young dog.

herbal medicine

Nettles and Parsley are beneficial, and may be administered either as infusions or chopped and added to food. Black-berry fruits – including Bramble, Bilberry, Elderberry and Black grapes – are beneficial either individually or combined; these may also be given as infusions or in the form of dietary supplements.

Bach flowers

Hornbeam is a strengthening remedy for the weary and weak.

minor therapies

biochemical tissue salts

Calc. phos., Nat. mur. and Ferr. phos. (all given in chronic dosage) help to increase red-blood-cell production and energy levels.

Chinese medicine

Dates, mung beans, spinach and shiitake mushrooms are the Chinese food remedies for anaemia. The following should be given (amounts depend on the size of dog): 1–3 tsps of chopped dates on alternate days; 1–3 tsps of sprouted mung beans daily; one to three chopped spinach leaves daily; and 1–3 tsps of chopped shiitake mushrooms daily.

crystals and gems

Ruby (liquid-gem remedy) may be given by mouth or added to water.

supplements

Food and supplements rich in iron and B-complex vitamins are beneficial for red-blood-cell production. Liver, Brewer's yeast, kelp, royal jelly and green vegetables are ideal. Giving extra Vitamin C is on a regular basis is also advisable.

lymphadenopathy

The lymphatic system is the body's 'drainage system', and the lymph glands act as detoxifying points along the route. Although linked with the circulation in general, the lymphatic system has its own set of diseases. Lymphoma is one of these (see pages 113–14); the second – more common – problem is lymphadenopathy, or non-cancerous enlargement of the lymph glands, which is usually caused by infection.

Signs and symptoms One or more enlarged and hardened lymph glands; general malaise.

homoeopathy

The following will be beneficial (all in chronic dosage): Baryta carb. for lymph-gland enlargement in a young or elderly dog; Calc. fluor. for very hard lymph glands, which almost feel like stones; and Conium mac. for hard glands in a weak dog (especially with incontinence and weak hindlegs). Phytolacca is effective for enlarged throat glands, and for inflamed mammary lymph glands in a bitch.

herbal medicine

Echinacea or Phytolacca may be given as infusions. 5 ml (1 tsp) Seaweed shredded in 10 ml (2 tsps) Apple cider can also be applied to enlarged lymph glands, especially if the glands feel hot and are painful.

minor therapies

crystals and gems

Topaz (liquid-gem remedy) may be given by mouth or added to water.

endocrine system

This is the network of glands producing the hormones that control body processes and metabolism. The most important glands in this system are the adrenal, thyroid and pituitary glands, and the areas of the pancreas that produce insulin. Diseases of these glands are difficult to control or to cure, and often need lifelong treatment. Although natural medicines may not be adequate on their own to effect cures or to give control of glandular problems, they are often an invaluable part of treatment. With dedicated care from the owner, a diabetic dog, for example, can lead a long and happy life.

diabetes mellitus

This condition results from a deficiency of the hormone insulin – which is needed to transfer glucose from the blood into body tissues – causing the body to become 'starved' of glucose. Diabetes can be caused by pancreatic disease and damage, and by the misuse of drugs such as steroids and hormones. Regular injections of insulin may be required, as natural medicines do not always cure diabetes, but the medicines are effective and can significantly reduce the need for injections.

Signs and symptoms Excessive thirst and hunger, weight loss, lethargy and cataracts (see page 71).

aromatherapy
Eucalyptus, Juniper and Lemon essential oils will all be beneficial when used for massage.

homoeopathy
Syzygium and Iris. vers. should be given in chronic dosage (continued dosage may vary from this: ask your vet for further advice).

herbal medicine
Oak bark, Olive root and Haricot-bean pods all make suitable infusions.

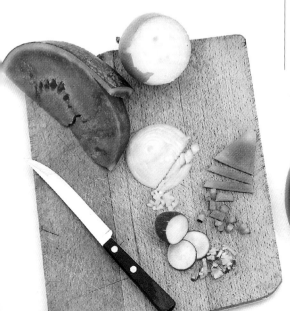

Watermelon peel, radish and onion are the food remedies advised in Chinese medicine for diabetes mellitus. These should be given as infusions for the best results.

Bach flowers
Hornbeam and Olive will help to alleviate lethargy and weakness.

minor therapies
biochemical tissue salts
Nat. mur. and Nat. sulph. may be alternated (both in chronic dosage).
Chinese medicine
Ginseng may be given in tablet form (50 mg daily), or as ¼ tsp of the diced root daily. Watermelon peel, radish and onion may also be given as daily infusions.
crystals and gems
Diamond (liquid-gem remedy) may be given by mouth or added to water.

natural therapies halve injections

Poppy was a middle-aged King Charles spaniel with middle-aged spread. However, her owner had recently noticed a distinct weight loss – despite Poppy being more hungry and thirsty than usual – and diabetes was diagnosed.

Poppy was given daily insulin injections, but the quantity required was increasing regularly and so her owner sought the help of natural medicines. She lived a long way away, making acupuncture impracticable, but I prescribed massage with Juniper and Lemon, Syzygium (homoeopathic remedy: chronic dosage) and the Bach flower Olive (twice daily). Six months later, Poppy's insulin dosage had been halved.

hypothyroidism

The thyroid glands are responsible for control of the body's metabolism. Hypothyroidism, a condition involving an underactivity of the thyroid gland, leads to a slowing down of the metabolism, affecting almost every body process. The cause may remain unknown – despite investigation – but is generally a form of inflammation of the thyroid gland (lymphocytic thyroiditis). Pituitary damage can also lead to hypothyroidism.

Signs and symptoms Obesity, lethargy, hair loss, lowered body temperature (the dog will look for warmth), and a slow heart rate.

homoeopathy
Flor de piedra and Thyroidinum should both be given in chronic dosage; if continued in the longer term, the dosage may need to change (consult your vet for further advice).

herbal medicine
Seaweed and Garlic (1–3 tsps daily, depending on the size of dog) may be added to food.

Bach flowers
Hornbeam and Olive are ideal remedies for lack of energy.

minor therapies
biochemical tissue salts
Nat. mur. (chronic dosage) helps to regulate body fluids.
Chinese medicine
Seaweed and kelp may both be given as infusions.

Cushing's disease
This condition – which is the opposite of Addison's disease (see below) – is caused by an overproduction of steroids by the adrenal glands. The reason for this is often unknown, although tumours of the adrenal or pituitary gland may be a factor.

Signs and symptoms Increased thirst and hunger, muscle stretching and weakness, alopecia (see pages 62–3), predisposition to skin infections, abdominal swelling and lethargy.

homoeopathy
Cortisone nosode and ACTH nosode (both in chronic dosage) will help to relieve the symptoms of this condition.

herbal medicine
Dandelion, Nettle, Watercress and Parsley may be given as infusions.

Bach flowers
Hornbeam and Olive will both help the 'weariness' and lethargy of Cushing's disease.

minor therapies
biochemical tissue salts
Nat. mur. (given in chronic dosage) will be beneficial.

Addison's disease
This is an underactivity of the adrenal glands, leading to a deficiency of the body's natural steroid production. It can become very serious, and a dog can collapse and even die as his or her steroid level falls. The cause may be unknown, although adrenal tumours, inflammations or thrombosis may be responsible. If long-term drug therapy with steroids is suddenly stopped, symptoms of Addison's disease can also be precipitated.

Signs and symptoms Muscle tremors, vomiting (see page 97), diarrhoea (see page 102), significant weight loss, an increased thirst and eventual collapse.

herbal medicine
Dandelion, Nettle, Watercress and Parsley essential oils will all be beneficial if given as infusions.

Bach flowers
Rock rose should be administered to alleviate acute symptoms, at a rate of one drop every 10 minutes for two hours.

minor therapies
biochemical tissue salts
Nat. mur. (chronic dose) is helpful.
Chinese medicine
Cloves and dates are the suggested food remedies in Chinese medicine: ¼ tsp of grated cloves and 1–3 tsps of chopped dates (depending on the size of the dog) should be added to food daily.

musculo-skeletal system

This system consists of the muscles, bones, joints, tendons and ligaments, which give the body shape and enable it to move. They are the parts that tend to suffer most from mechanical wear and tear, injury and inflammation, and can also be very difficult to put right once they have gone wrong.

Of the natural therapies available, acupuncture and T-touch massage will help any disorder of the musculo-skeletal system; osteopathy and chiropractic have also been found to be beneficial in many cases.

arthritis

Arthritis, or joint inflammation, is mainly a problem of the older dog. This form of arthritis – called osteoarthritis – is caused by general wear and tear, but joint inflammation in younger dogs also occurs occasionally due to injury, infection or disease of the immune system.

Signs and symptoms Stiffness and pain in the arthritic joints, resulting in persistent lameness.

aromatherapy

Juniper, Birch, Pine, Thyme, Terebinth and Rosemary may all be used for gentle massage.

homoeopathy

The following may all be given (in chronic dosage unless stated): Acid. sal. for rheumatic pains in 'small' joints; Apis mel. (acute dosage) for a sudden, hot swelling of the joint and a taut, shiny appearance; Bryonia for a dry, stiff 'cracking' joint that worsens with movement; Calc. carb. for a stiff, overweight, lethargic dog; Causticum for a stiff, old dog who may also be becoming senile; Caulophyllum for arthritis in knee, hock and other 'small' joints; and Rhus tox., the 'classic' remedy for typical arthritic symptoms that worsen in cold, damp weather and are more severe after rest.

herbal medicine

Feverfew, Devil's claw, Comfrey, Cleavers, Burdock, Yarrow, Alfalfa, White-willow bark, Yucca and the 'green-leaf' herbs (Nettle, Parsley, Dandelion and Watercress) can all be given as infusions. Many are also available in tablet form – some in compatible combinations.

Added daily to a dog's diet, royal jelly – secreted by worker bees – and cod-liver-oil capsules can help to relieve arthritic pain (see also page 48).

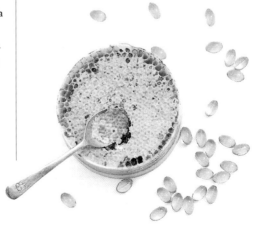

Bach flowers

Crabapple is an ideal cleansing remedy for toxins in the joints; Hornbeam will enhance strength.

acupuncture

Arthritis is particularly responsive to acupuncture.

minor therapies

biochemical tissue salts

Ferr. phos. (acute dosage) is suitable for sudden-onset, acute arthritis; Calc. fluor. (chronic dosage) for chronic arthritis.

Chinese medicine

Cinnamon (powdered) should be given (¼ tsp twice weekly). Royal jelly is beneficial: 100 mg per 23 kg (50 lb) body weight should be given daily.

crystals and gems

Ruby (liquid-gem remedy) may be given by mouth or added to water.

osteopathy and chiropractic

Some forms of arthritis – especially of the spine – greatly benefit from these forms of manipulation.

supplements

The following will all be effective: kelp; cider vinegar (5 ml [1 tsp] per 600 ml [1 pt] of drinking water); Vitamin C (250 mg–3 g, depending on the size of dog, daily); cod-liver oil (500 mg per 14 kg [30 lb] body weight, daily); green-lipped-mussel extract (at the recommended human dosage rate); B-complex vitamins (10–20 mg daily); and Vitamin E (100 iu daily). Chondroitin sulphate is available in proprietary form for animals: this should be administered according to the specific instructions supplied. Copper collars are also very beneficial for arthritis sufferers.

natural therapies prolong life

Prince was a 16-year-old, very stiff Shetland sheepdog who had several arthritic joints. He seemed to experience severe side-effects to the use of any conventional anti-inflammatory, painkilling drugs, and he was so stiff and in so much discomfort that euthanasia was the inevitable next step if natural medicines, as a last resort, could not help.

Fortunately there is an array of remedies for arthritis, and I chose those appropriate to Prince's symptoms. The stiffness was worse when resting, but eased when he got himself moving, and worsened in cold, damp weather: this indicated the homoeopathic remedy Rhus tox. (chronic dosage). Prince also had slight water retention, due to a mild heart problem. The 'green-leaf' herbs – Nettles, Parsley and Dandelion – were given as infusions: these act as gentle diuretics (that is, they remove excess fluid from the system), and also act as anti-arthritic agents. Prince was also fitted with a copper chain, an invaluable aid in relieving arthritic stiffness in very old dogs.

This combination of homoeopathy, herbs and copper resulted in a significant increase in Prince's mobility, as well as a substantial reduction in his discomfort. He died peacefully in his sleep a year later, just after reaching his 17th birthday. However, his owners were very pleased that he had been given some extra months of active life, and that the decision on euthanasia had never had to be made.

sprains and strains

Pulled muscles, inflamed tendons, stretched ligaments – a whole range of minor injuries falls under the heading of sprains and strains. Bandages are difficult to keep in place on dogs, so this usual human remedy is less appropriate, but natural medicines can help to promote a rapid recovery.

Signs and symptoms Lameness, pain and sometimes an obvious swelling of the affected area.

aromatherapy

Rosemary, Juniper or Birch may be massaged into the area.

homoeopathy

Arnica (acute dosage) should be given as soon as possible, followed by Ruta grav. (chronic dosage). Rhus tox. (chronic dosage) is beneficial for persistent lameness following a sprain or strain.

herbal medicine

Mallow may be given as infusions.

acupuncture

A course of this treatment is often rapidly effective.

minor therapies

Biochemical tissue salts

Ferr. phos. given alternately with Nat. phos. (both in acute dosage) is ideal for a recent sprain or strain; Mag. phos. alternating with Calc. phos. (chronic dosage) is suitable for a longstanding problem.

T-touch massage

A course of this form of massage will help to relieve the pain of a sprain or strain injury, and will promote healing and a quick recovery.

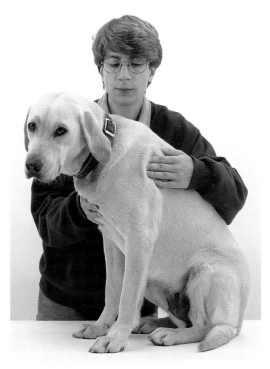

In T-touch massage, small circular movements are made at random over the dog's body. This process is said to generate specific brainwave patterns, instilling calmness and thereby preventing overuse of the injured limb so that natural healing can occur (see also pages 30–1).

joint dislocation

The hips and shoulders of a dog are the joints that are most likely to dislocate through accidents, but small breeds are also predisposed to dislocation of the patella (kneecap). Physical replacement of the joint by a vet will be necessary, but natural remedies will help to prevent redislocation (this may occur due to damage caused to the ligaments).

Signs and symptoms A dislocation causes obvious and sometimes dramatic lameness; the joint may be visibly misshapen.

homoeopathy

Rhus tox. and Ruta grav. should be given alternately (in chronic dosage).

minor therapies

biochemical tissue salts

Calc. fluor. and Calc. phos. (both in chronic dosage) should be given alternately to relieve pain.

supplements

Vitamin C (250 mg–3 g daily, depending on the size of the dog) will help to promote rapid healing of the damaged tissue in the joint.

bone fracture

Bone fractures may be 'closed' (with unbroken skin), or 'open' (the broken bone penetrates the skin). They are also classified as simple (one straightforward break) or comminuted (in several pieces). Fractures are usually caused by accidents, but can be spontaneous in thin or brittle bones. A fracture needs immediate treatment – sometimes with surgery – but natural medicines can play an important role in recovery.

Signs and symptoms Instant, obvious pain and lameness; the broken bone ends may be heard grating, or may be visible, sticking out of the skin (in an 'open' fracture).

homoeopathy

If given immediately, Arnica will minimize bruising and tissue damage. Symphytum will accelerate the subsequent healing process (both to be given in acute dosage).

herbal medicine

Comfrey, given daily for two weeks as an infusion, will greatly assist the healing process.

acupuncture

A course of this treatment often produces excellent results.

minor therapies

biochemical tissue salts

Calc. fluor. may be alternated with Calc. phos. (both in chronic dosage).

supplements

Vitamin C (250 mg–3 g daily) will promote healing.

hip dysplasia

This is a developmental defect of the hip joints, and is especially common in the German shepherd, labrador and retriever. One or both hips become malformed, leading to arthritis (see pages 83–4) and sometimes partial dislocation. The condition may be evident at a few months of age, or later in life. It may be aggravated by a poor diet, and possibly by over-exercising a puppy. **Signs and symptoms** Some dogs suffer from only mild symptoms (a 'rolling' gait while walking and hindleg stiffness); others may be incapacitated and require surgery.

homoeopathy

The following are suitable remedies (all in chronic dosage): Colocynth; Calc. carb. for a heavily built dog; and Calc. phos. for a lighter, thinner dog.

herbal medicine

Alfalfa, Burdock, Comfrey and White-willow bark may be given as infusions, or in tablet form.

acupuncture

A course of this treatment will often produce excellent results in a case of hip dysplasia.

minor therapies

biochemical tissue salts

Calc. fluor. should be alternated with Calc. phos. (chronic dosage).

osteopathy and chiropractic

A course of either treatment will help to relieve pain.

supplements

The following are all recommended: Vitamin C (250 mg–3 g, depending on size, daily); B-complex vitamins (10–20 mg daily); and Vitamin E (100 mg daily). Cider vinegar may be added to drinking water, at a rate of 5 ml (1 tsp) per 600 ml (1 pt).

disc protrusion

Often known as a 'slipped disc', this follows degeneration of a disc, which acts as a shock absorber between two spinal vertebrae. The disc begins to press on the spinal cord, and the result can be severe (sometimes permanent) weakness and paralysis. Breeds with long backs (such as the dachshund) are prone to disc protrusion. The condition may occur unexpectedly, or following injury. **Signs and symptoms** Sudden back or neck pain, with general weakness or paralysis.

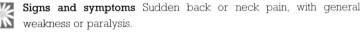

homoeopathy

Hypericum relieves nerve pain; Arnica reduces bruising; and Nux vomica relieves back pain (in acute dosage).

herbal medicine

Feverfew will ease the pain and is best given as fresh leaves, although these have a bitter taste (two to three leaves should be added to food twice daily). Comfrey may be given as an infusion for short periods. Skullcap with Valerian – also available in tablet form – will soothe and calm.

Bach flowers

Rescue Remedy will help to alleviate pain and shock.

acupuncture

Disc problems often respond well to a course of acupuncture.

minor therapies

biochemical tissue salts

Mag. phos. (acute dosage), followed by Calc. fluor. and Calc. phos. (given alternately, in chronic dosage), will help to relieve the pain.

Chinese medicine

Cinnamon is the recommended Chinese remedy: ¼ tsp, powdered, should be given daily.

crystals and gems

Sapphire (liquid-gem remedy) may be given by mouth or added to water.

spondylosis

This occurs when extra bone is laid down around the spinal vertebrae. The new bone may grow until it meets and fuses with an adjacent vertebra, causing stiffness, and it may press on the nerves leaving the spinal cord, interfering with nerve function.

Signs and symptoms An inflexible, painful spine; weakness or paralyis of one or more legs.

controlling spondylosis

Herman was a rottweiler of huge proportions. Although he had been fit and well for most of his life, middle age was catching up with him and, at seven years old, he had developed cervial spondylosis (basically a stiff neck, although the growth of extra bone in the adjacent vertebra made the condition a potentially serious one).

Six osteopathy sessions improved the stiffness considerably, and Herman also went swimming in a special hydrotherapy pool for dogs. I then gave him six acupuncture sessions, at weekly intervals, which had an even greater effect. Herman now has occasional osteopathic manipulations, and acupuncture therapy every two months, and so far continues to do well.

homoeopathy

Hypericum (chronic dosage) is effective for the pain caused by the pressure on nerves; Causticum is useful for 'tearing' pains and stiffness in an older dog.

acupuncture

This therapy is often very beneficial.

minor therapies

biochemical tissue salts

Calc. fluor. should be administered alternately with Calc. phos. (both in chronic dosage).

osteopathy and chiropractic

Both of these treatments are helpful in most cases.

CDRM

Chronic degenerative radiculo myelopathy is caused by a degeneration of the nerves supplying the hindquarters, resulting in gradual paralysis and loss of sensation. It often affects the German shepherd. This condition is painless, but many dogs ultimately have their lives ended because of the distress caused by the symptoms.

Signs and symptoms Loss of hindquarter strength and swaying (eventually the hindleg muscles waste away, making walking impossible), and incontinence.

aromatherapy
Juniper and Elder may be massaged around the hindquarters.

homoeopathy
Conium mac. and Plumb. met. (both to be given in chronic dosage) will increase strength in the hindquarters.

acupuncture
CDRM may respond to a course of acupuncture treatment.

minor therapies
biochemical tissue salts
Kali phos. (chronic dosage) may help.
Chinese medicine
Cherries (three to six, depending on the size of dog, daily) are advised.
crystals and gems
Ruby (liquid remedy) may be given.
supplements
Vitamin C (250 mg–3 g) and blackcurrant-seed oil (500 mg) should be given daily.

Feverfew has a natural anti-inflammatory action, and will help to reduce swelling and discomfort.

myositis

Myositis (muscle inflammation) is a painful condition. It may be caused by infection, injury or disease of the immune system.

Signs and symptoms The affected muscle may become swollen, and hard, and will be tender to the touch.

homoeopathy
Aconite (acute dosage) is effective if given early, followed by Rhus tox. alternating with Bryonia (chronic dosage). Causticum (chronic dosage) will help any remaining stiffness.

herbal medicine
Feverfew is best given as fresh leaves (one to three leaves, three times daily), although the dog may object to the bitter taste.

minor therapies
biochemical tissue salts
Ferr. phos. (acute dosage) will be helpful if given at an early stage; this should be followed by Nat. phos. alternated with Mag. phos. (chronic dosage).
Chinese medicine
Black soybeans may be given as infusions.

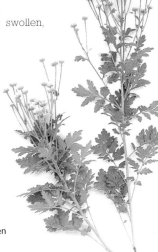

osteomyelitis

This is an infection that occurs within the bone. As antibiotics are not able to penetrate bone easily, an infection of this type can be very serious, and also extremely difficult to cure. Osteomyelitis could arise following a fracture (see page 86) or other kind of bone injury.

Signs and symptoms Pain, fever and swelling of the affected area; there may also be a discharge of pus. The dog will be obviously lame on the affected limb.

homoeopathy

Aconite (acute dosage) can be very effective if it is administered at an early stage – especially if fever is also present. Hepar sulph. (to be given in acute dosage) is the homoeopathic anti-infective remedy, and is suitable for use in a case of osteomyelitis. As the infection clears, Calc. carb. (for a heavy dog) and Calc. phos. (for a lighter dog) – both to be given in chronic dosage – will help to strengthen the bone.

minor therapies
biochemical tissue salts
Calc. fluor. should be alternated with Calc. phos. (chronic dosage). If the infection persists, Calc. sulph. (chronic dosage) should be added.

osteochondrosis

In this condition small flakes of cartilage peel away from the bone within a joint, causing pain and lameness. The shoulder joint is most commonly affected. Large breeds are more likely to suffer from osteochondrosis, and the condition is seen in young dogs, normally in the first two years. It may be related to dietary imbalance or to rapid growth in a large, heavy breed.

Signs and symptoms Lameness, with intense pain and an obvious swelling at the affected joint.

homoeopathy
The following are effective remedies (all in chronic dosage): Calc. carb. for a big-boned, heavy dog; Calc. phos. for a thinner, lighter dog; and Calc. fluor. to strengthen the joints.

acupuncture
This is a very beneficial therapy in the treatment of osteochondrosis.

minor therapies
biochemical tissue salts
Calc. fluor. should be alternated with Calc. phos.; Silica will be beneficial if thickening of the joint persists (all in chronic dosage).

Chinese medicine
Shiitake mushrooms are advised: 1–3 tsps (depending on the size of dog), chopped, should be given daily.

nervous system

This section covers diseases of the brain and nerves. Behavioural problems are dealt with separately (see pages 120–5).

The brain and nervous system are the command and control system for the body. From receiving information via sensory organs such as the eyes and ears, to organizing control of muscle contractions and regulating the beating of the heart, a dog's nervous system is integral to his or her overall body function.

convulsions

Convulsions, or fits, are very frightening to watch. Epilepsy is caused by abnormal brain activity; other causes of fits include ingestion of poisons (such as anti-freeze), infection (such as distemper – see page 118), metabolic disorders (such as diabetes mellitus – see pages 80–1), injury or a brain tumour. A dog in a fit should be kept as quiet as possible, ideally in a darkened room.

Signs and symptoms In a non-epileptic fit the dog will have muscle tremors, rigidity, loss of balance and muscle spasms. An epileptic fit is similar, but there may be confusion before and after the fit. Weakness, restlessness and a need to eat or drink are also typical.

aromatherapy
Lavender, Sweet marjoram and Camomile may be given by infusion, either after a fit or between fits.

homoeopathy
Cocculus (chronic dosage) is a preventive remedy for convulsions. Tarentula hisp. (chronic dosage) is helpful for a dog who remains 'twitchy' after or between fits. The following may be given after a fit: Belladonna (acute dosage) if the pupils remain dilated; Cicuta virosa if the head is stretched back or to the side during the fit (acute dosage after the fit, then chronic dosage); Bufo (chronic dosage) if fits start during sleep; and Stramonium (acute dosage) if the dog falls to the left side.

herbal medicine
Skullcap with Valerian may be given either as infusions or in tablet form. Hops, Rosemary, or Valerian with Melissa (Lemon balm) may also be used as infusions.

Bach flowers
Vervain and Chestnut bud will help.

minor therapies
biochemical tissue salts
Kali phos. (chronic dosage) may be given.
Chinese medicine
Dates (1–3 tsps, depending on the size of dog) may be given daily.
crystals and gems
Diamond (liquid-gem remedy) may be given by mouth or added to water.

neuritis

Inflammation of a nerve, or group of nerves, will lead to excessive discomfort in the area of tissue supplied by that nerve or nerves. For instance, a persistent localized itchiness of the skin may be caused by inflammation of the nerve supplying that part of the skin. Possible causes are injuries (including surgical wounds), infections, pressure (for example, that caused by a 'trapped' nerve), or a tumour.

Signs and symptoms Persistent localized pain or irritation, resulting in constant licking, scratching or biting at the affected area.

aromatherapy
Lavender may be massaged into the skin at or near the affected area.

homoeopathy
The following are helpful (all to be given in chronic dosage): Passiflora is a general soothing remedy; Chamomilla is suitable for an irritable and snappy dog; and Hypericum is ideal where there is physical damage at a nerve ending, such as at the site of a cut or bruise.

herbal medicine
Oats or Passiflora may be given by infusion.

Bach flowers
Star of Bethlehem may be beneficial.

minor therapies
biochemical tissue salts
Mag. phos. (chronic dosage) will assist in relieving the symptoms.
crystals and gems
Sapphire (liquid remedy) may help.

encephalitis and meningitis

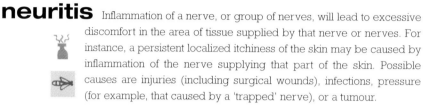

These serious diseases both affect the brain. Encephalitis is an inflammation within the brain tissue; meningitis is an inflammation of the tissues around the brain. Causes include bacterial or viral infections, or a tumour.

Signs and symptoms Pain (demonstrated by pressing of the head against solid objects), behavioural changes, hindleg paralysis, swaying, falling and fits.

aromatherapy
Lavender may be given by massage.

homoeopathy
Belladonna may be given if the pupils are dilated; Cuprum met. for muscle twitchings; and Stramonium if the dog falls to the left (all in acute dosage).

herbal medicine
Sage, Thyme, Marjoram, Rice and Skullcap may all be administered in the form of infusions.

Bach flowers
Rock rose may help to alleviate the symptoms of both conditions.

chorea

Chorea is an involuntary twitching of the muscles. It usually occurs in dogs following distemper infection (see page 118), but can also be caused by poisoning, or by a tumour in the brain.

Signs and symptoms Uncontrollable twitching, particularly of the limbs and facial muscles.

aromatherapy

Lavender should be given by massage.

homoeopathy

The following are helpful (all in chronic dosage): Agaricus for classic 'distemper' chorea symptoms; Causticum for a dog who is old and stiff; and Conium, especially if the hindquarters are weakened.

herbal medicine

Skullcap combined with Valerian may be administered either as infusions or in tablet form; and Rue, Oats, Rosemary or Lily-of-the-valley may be used as infusions.

Bach flowers

Scleranthus may help to control the symptoms.

minor therapies

biochemical tissue salts
Kali phos. (chronic dosage) may be beneficial.

Chinese medicine
Chicken-egg yolks (one to three, twice weekly) should be given.

crystals and gems
Diamond (liquid remedy) may help.

homoeopathy eases symptoms

Bernard had rather an unoriginal name – he was a St Bernard. This large breed is not long-lived, and at seven Bernard was showing signs of old age: his hindquarters were weak, and he had a continuous tremor in his hindlegs. The homoeopathic remedy Conium mac. – from the poisonous water-hemlock plant – fitted these symptoms, and I prescribed a chronic dosage.

Although never regaining great strength in his hindlegs, the tremors lessened significantly, and Bernard managed to keep his hindquarters in working order until his death a year later.

Although natural medicines may not be able to eliminate chorea entirely, they can help to reduce the twitching of the muscles.

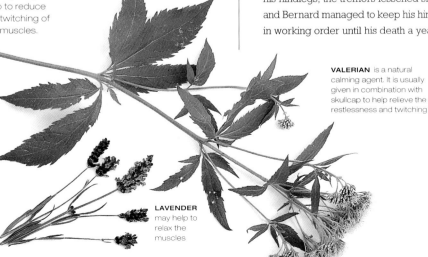

VALERIAN is a natural calming agent. It is usually given in combination with skullcap to help relieve the restlessness and twitching

LAVENDER may help to relax the muscles

digestive system

A dog's digestive system starts – naturally enough – in the mouth, where it includes the teeth and any associated gum and dental disorders, as well as abnormalities of the salivary glands. The stomach and intestines, and all their possible problems, come next: due to the scavenging habits of many dogs, vomiting after the ingestion of unsuitable food is a particularly common disorder. The liver and pancreas are also closely associated with digestion and are prone to a number of different conditions. The digestive system ends at the rectum, and includes common lower-bowel problems such as constipation and diarrhoea.

dental disease

As a dog's diet is low in sugary foods, the likelihood of dental decay – as often occurs in humans – is small. However, the teeth do become diseased in other ways: for example, due to infection following damage, or because of gum erosion. Any necessary dental work will be assisted by the remedies listed below.

Signs and symptoms Obvious pain when eating, drooling, loose or visibly damaged teeth and bad breath.

homoeopathy
The following may all be used (in chronic dosage): Hepar sulph. will help to fight infection; Merc. sol. controls bad breath and excessive salivation; and Hypericum has a soothing effect and helps to relieves the pain of diseased teeth.

minor therapies
biochemical tissue salts

Calc. fluor. (administered in chronic dosage) is an excellent preventive remedy that has a dual role: it helps to strengthen the teeth, thereby increasing their resistance to infection and decay.

salivary cyst

A swelling in the facial area is often assumed to be an abscess, but a saliva-filled cyst is another possibility. The reason for such cysts is unknown. Surgical drainage is normally required, and may need to be repeated if the cyst subsequently refills.

Signs and symptoms The appearance of a soft facial swelling that increases in size.

homoeopathy
The following are all useful remedies: Apis mel. is helpful for a soft swelling that 'pits' on pressure; Phytolacca is suitable for a firm swelling; and Silicea may be used at a later stage when the swelling has hardened (all to be given in chronic dosage).

gingivitis and stomatitis

Gingivitis (or gum inflammation) and stomatitis (inflammation of the mouth lining) often occur together. They may be associated with diseased teeth or result from infection, poisoning (for example by lead), kidney disease (see page 104) or immune-system disease. Dental treatment should be followed by a raw-food-based diet containing hard, crunchy foods.

Signs and symptoms Reddened gums, mouth ulcers, pain on eating, bad breath and excessive drooling.

aromatherapy

Terebinth and Lavender essential oils may be used for massage.

homoeopathy

The following remedies will provide symptomatic relief (acute dosage in the early stages; chronic dosage for a longstanding case): Acid. nit. or Borax for gingivitis with mouth ulcers; Belladonna for a very red mouth and a feverish patient; Merc. cor. for pain and profuse salivation; and Phosphorus for bleeding gums.

herbal medicine

Echinacea, Myrrh and Goldenseal, in the form of a tincture, may be applied directly to the gums and mouth. Sage and Rosemary may be given as infusions.

minor therapies

biochemical tissue salts

Calc. sulph. (in acute dosage) is appropriate where the gums are swollen and bleeding.

Chinese medicine

Persimmon (sharon fruit) and star fruit may be beneficial; ⅓ to one fruit should be given daily.

crystals and gems

Emerald (liquid-gem remedy) may be given by mouth or added to water.

resolving gingivitis

Some dogs just will not brush their teeth regularly, and Dennis the dachshund was no exception to this rule. Or, rather, he refused to let his owner brush his teeth for him. Neither would he gnaw bones, nor eat healthy hard, crunchy foods such as raw vegetables. In short, Dennis had only himself to blame for the painful gingivitis from which he was suffering when I first saw him. He had already received dental treatment, involving tooth-scaling and then polishing, but the sore gums remained, together with a tendency to dribble saliva and a marked – and very anti-social – halitosis. I prescribed the homoeopathic remedy Merc. cor. (chronic dosage) to soothe the sore gums and reduce the salivation, together with the herb Goldenseal as a tincture to be applied to the gums – whether Dennis liked it or not!

The improvement in the symptoms after a short period of treatment was considerable, and Dennis even became so accustomed to the application of the herbal tincture that he gave in and allowed his owner to start brushing his teeth. The gingivitis has not recurred since.

pharyngitis

Pharyngitis is, essentially, a sore throat – and everyone knows how painful that can be. The condition in dogs may occur due to viral, bacterial or fungal infections, after swallowing certain irritant poisons, or because of a foreign body that has become lodged in the dog's pharynx (throat).

Signs and symptoms Persistent coughing, retching, lack of appetite, and enlargement of the lymph glands beneath the jaw.

aromatherapy
Bergamot, Hyssop, Sage and Thyme will all provide relief when gently massaged into the throat area.

homoeopathy
The following relieve soreness (all in chronic dosage): Baryta carb. for a young dog with swollen lymph glands; Lachesis for an inflamed, purplish throat; and Phytolacca for a painful throat with enlarged lymph glands.

herbal medicine
Echinacea tincture will soothe the throat, and should given by mouth three times daily.

Bach flowers
Star of Bethlehem will help to relax a 'tense' throat.

minor therapies
biochemical tissue salts
Calc. phos. is suitable for pharyngitis with tonsillitis; Calc. sulph. for a painful, ulcerated throat; and Ferr. phos. for pharyngitis with laryngitis.
Chinese medicine
The following are suggested: lemon juice (5 ml [1 tsp]) mixed with a little honey twice daily; and star fruit (⅓ to one fruit daily).
crystals and gems
Sapphire (liquid remedy) may help.

Fruits and herbs are among the remedies most often used to treat digestive disorders. Those shown here will all provide rapid relief for the discomfort of pharyngitis.

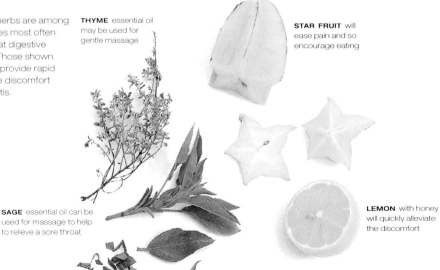

THYME essential oil may be used for gentle massage

STAR FRUIT will ease pain and so encourage eating

SAGE essential oil can be used for massage to help to relieve a sore throat

LEMON with honey will quickly alleviate the discomfort

vomiting

Occasional vomiting in dogs is not unusual. Common causes include eating inappropriate foods, infections, foreign bodies, intestinal abnormalities, and liver, pancreatic or kidney disease. After vomiting, food should be withheld for 24 hours, and then a bland diet given.

Signs and symptoms Unmissable! If a dog is vomiting frequently, vomiting blood or vomiting with other acute symptoms, he or she must be examined by a vet as soon as possible.

aromatherapy

Mint, Lavender and Tarragon may all be either used for massage or administered via a diffuser.

homoeopathy

The following may be helpful (acute dosage for severe vomiting; chronic dosage for persistent vomiting): Arsen. alb. for vomiting with diarrhoea that may be related to poisoning; Apomorphine for repeated vomiting, often occurring as soon as food has been swallowed; Ipecac. for intermittent but recurrent vomiting with a great deal of retching; Nux vomica for post-operative vomiting and vomiting after eating unsuitable foods; and Phosphorus for vomiting that occurs shortly after eating.

herbal medicine

Infusions of Gentian root, St John's wort or Peppermint will all help to alleviate the symptoms.

minor therapies

biochemical tissue salts

The following are all suitable (in acute dosage for severe vomiting; or chronic dosage for a longstanding problem): Ferr. phos. for vomiting of undigested food; Kali mur. for vomiting of thick mucus, especially after eating particularly fatty food; Nat. phos. for sour, acid vomit and an irritable patient; and Nat. sulph. for vomited bile.

Chinese medicine

Fennel seeds are recommended to relieve vomiting: 1–3 tsps (depending on the size of the dog) should be added to food daily.

crystals and gems

Emerald (liquid-gem remedy) may be given by mouth or added to water.

resolving a case of vomiting

Patrick had only one vice: gluttony. He was a portly beagle who lived life on one principle: if it looks good, eat it. On one occasion Patrick used this principle to consume two weeks' supply of his usual dog food – which had been accidentally left within reach – at a single sitting. His body was now trying to make amends by returning the food to the outside world.

I put Patrick on an acute dosage of the homoeopathic remedy Nux vomica, along with an occasional 5 ml (1 tsp) of Peppermint infusion, a herbal agent used to calm digestion. Within two hours, the vomiting had stopped and Patrick looked a happy beagle once again.

pyloric stenosis

 This is a constriction of the opening to the stomach, which prevents the stomach from functioning normally. The cause may be unknown, or may be a congenital abnormality. Surgery is often required, but the remedies outlined below will also help.

Signs and symptoms Persistent and often particularly forceful ('projectile') vomiting.

homoeopathy

Nux vomica alternated with Staphisagria (chronic dosage) will assist in restoring normal stomach function. Ornithogallum tincture may be given (one drop three times daily). If surgery is needed, Silicea (chronic dosage) will minimize scarring.

gastric torsion

In this potentially life-threatening condition, fermentation causes gas to fill the stomach, which then twists round on itself, sealing the gas inside. The stomach continues to expand as more gas is produced, causing increasing pain, shock and pressure on other organs. Urgent veterinary treatment – possibly to pass a tube down into the stomach, or to carry out surgery – will be required.

Signs and symptoms Abdominal swelling and pain.

homoeopathy

The following are all good remedies: Ornithogallum tincture and Colocynth (both in acute dosage); and Nux moschata (chronic dosage) after an attack to help prevent recurrence.

foreign bodies

 Dogs swallow all kinds of objects. Some do pass safely through the digestive system – I once saw a tiny Tibetan terrier puppy who had swallowed a hat pin half as long as himself, which came out at the other end without causing harm – but other objects become lodged in the oesophagus, stomach or the intestines. If a foreign body is obstructing the intestine, surgery will be necessary; in other cases, the object may eventually pass through, or be vomited up.

Signs and symptoms Vomiting, little or no passage of faeces, abdominal pain and lethargy.

homoeopathy

Colchicum is suitable for an intestinal blockage; Ornithogallum tincture for the stomach (both in acute dosage).

minor therapies

crystals and gems

Emerald (liquid-gem remedy) may be given by mouth or added to water.

colic

Some dogs – mainly small breeds – are prone to bouts of colic. Loud rumbling and gurgling noises can be heard as gases build up in the intestines, and muscular spasms of the intestinal wall can cause pain and discomfort. Colic may be caused by an imbalanced diet, or a dietary allergy, but often there is no obvious reason.

Signs and symptoms General uneasiness and an arched back. The dog may stare at his or flanks, whine with pain or fright, and make straining attempts to defecate.

aromatherapy
Cinnamon and Caraway essential oils may be used for frequent massage over the stomach area.

homoeopathy
The following are helpful (all in chronic dosage): Carbo vegetabilis for a flatulent dog who may be weak or have collapsed; Colchicum for a dog who will not eat, and may be vomiting and/or have diarrhoea, with a bloated abdomen; and Colocynth for a dog with an arched back, whose pain comes in waves.

minor therapies
biochemical tissue salts
Mag. phos. and Nat. sulph. may be given alternately (acute dosage).

intussusception

In this potentially serious condition, the intestine telescopes into itself as a result of excessive muscular movements of the bowel wall. This causes an obstruction, which can be potentially very serious if not dealt with rapidly. Surgery is normally required, but in the early stages natural remedies can be successful. Common causes of intussusception are an acute bout of diarrhoea (see page 102) or an infestation of parasitic worms (see page 117).

Puppies are particularly prone to intestinal-worm infestations, and – due to their immature digestive systems – are also prone to diarrhoea. For these reasons, intussusception is more commonly seen in puppies than in adult dogs; because of their young age, the condition can be life-threatening.

Signs and symptoms Persistent vomiting and diarrhoea, straining and an abdomen that is painful to touch.

homoeopathy
Colchicum and Nux vomica should be administered alternately (in acute dosages) to relieve muscle spasm.

minor therapies
crystals and gems
Emerald (liquid-gem remedy) may be given by mouth or added to water.

liver disease

The liver has a variety of functions: these include producing enzymes needed for digestion, controlling the distribution of nutrients, and detoxifying poisons. Liver disease may be acute or chronic. Causes include infections, poisoning, tumours, bile-duct obstruction and disease of the immune system.

Signs and symptoms Vomiting, weight loss, lethargy, ascites (see page 77) and jaundice.

aromatherapy

Mint with Rosemary may be used for massage in acute liver disease; Wild marjoram with rosemary in chronic liver disease.

homoeopathy

The following remedies are effective (all in chronic dosage): Carduus for cirrhosis, a swollen liver and ascites; Chelidonium if jaundice is evident; Lycopodium for digestive problems and flatulence; Nux vomica for persistent digestive upsets; and Phosphorus for pain and vomiting.

herbal medicine

One of the following herbs – Blue flag, Centaury, Southernwood, Dandelion and Yellow dock – may be given by infusion.

minor therapies

biochemical tissue salts

Nat. sulph. (chronic dosage) may be beneficial.

Chinese medicine

Add one or two diced plums (depending on the size of the dog) and 1–3 tsps each of chopped hickory and kohl rabi to food daily.

pancreatitis

There are three types of pancreatic disease in dogs: diabetes mellitus (see pages 80–1), pancreatic insufficiency (where digestive enzymes are lacking: enzyme supplementation and a low-fat diet are normally necessary), and pancreatitis, an inflammatory condition that may follow steroid use and can be fatal. Emergency surgery may be needed; otherwise the following remedies will help.

Signs and symptoms Pain, fever, vomiting, diarrhoea (see page 102) and lack of appetite.

homoeopathy

Phosphorus and Iris vers. (acute dosage) are both suitable remedies.

herbal medicine

Gentian may be given as an infusion.

minor therapies

biochemical tissue salts

Nat. phos. should be given alternately with Ferr. phos. (acute dosage).

crystals and gems

Topaz (liquid remedy) may be given.

constipation

Dogs generally suffer much less frequently from constipation than we do. However, it is an occasional problem, and is no less uncomfortable for them than it is for us. Constipation may be caused by too many cooked bones, or by insufficient fibre in the diet (this may be rectified by adding raw vegetables and cereals to food – see pages 41–5). Constipation may also result from an enlarged or constricted lower bowel, or from polyps or tumours in the bowel.

Signs and symptoms Obvious straining to defecate, the production of thin, flattened faeces (or none at all) and long periods between bowel movements.

homoeopathy

The following should all be given in chronic dosage: Calc. carb. for large, chalky stools (especially after eating bones); Nux vomica for post-operative constipation, or after overeating; Sepia for constipation associated with liver problems; and Silicea where the stool is almost passed, but then recedes into the rectum (often known as the 'shy-stool' syndrome).

herbal medicine

Rhubarb can be used as an infusion, or a small amount may be added directly to the diet. Frangula bark, used as an infusion, is a gentle and efficacious remedy.

Bach flowers

Crabapple is known as the cleansing remedy, and is appropriate in a case of constipation.

minor therapies

biochemical tissue salts

The following may also be used (all to be administered in chronic dosage): Calc. fluor. for a completely inactive bowel; Kali mur. for a bout of constipation following overeating or the consumption of rich food; and Nat. mur. for constipation alternating with diarrhoea. Nat. phos. and Nat. sulph. may also be given alternately for persistent constipation.

Chinese medicine

White radish is helpful: one to three of these (depending on the size of the dog), chopped, should be mixed with food daily.

crystals and gems

Ruby (liquid-gem remedy) may be given by mouth or added to water.

supplements

Bran, dried fruit and psyllium husks are particularly effective as part of a high-fibre diet. Liquid paraffin may be used as a lubricating and loosening agent, and often provides rapid relief from constipation. However, it does prevent the Vitamins A, D, E and K from being absorbed by the body, and persistent use will result in vitamin deficiency, so always consult your vet before giving it to your dog for any length of time.

diarrhoea

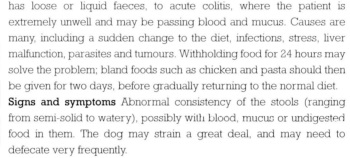

This can vary from mild symptoms, where a dog simply has loose or liquid faeces, to acute colitis, where the patient is extremely unwell and may be passing blood and mucus. Causes are many, including a sudden change to the diet, infections, stress, liver malfunction, parasites and tumours. Withholding food for 24 hours may solve the problem; bland foods such as chicken and pasta should then be given for two days, before gradually returning to the normal diet.

Signs and symptoms Abnormal consistency of the stools (ranging from semi-solid to watery), possibly with blood, mucus or undigested food in them. The dog may strain a great deal, and may need to defecate very frequently.

aromatherapy

Cinnamon may be given by massage.

homoeopathy

The following will be helpful (acute dosage for sudden diarrhoea; chronic dosage for long-term diarrhoea): Aloe for flatulence and mucus; Arsen. alb. for food poisoning (with vomiting); Chamomilla for green, frothy diarrhoea; Colocynth for diarrhoea with colicky pains and an arched back; Merc. sol. for loose stools but no pain; Phosphorus for straining, with mucus and/or blood; and Podophyllum for watery faeces.

herbal medicine

Arrowroot, Catechu, dried Bilberries, Meadowsweet, Plantain and Slippery elm may be given (Slippery elm is available as tablets; the others may be given as infusions).

Bach flowers

For stress-related diarrhoea, Impatiens is helpful for an irritable dog; Aspen for an anxious one.

minor therapies

biochemical tissue salts

The following are all beneficial (acute dosage for acute diarrhoea; chronic dosage for longstanding diarrhoea): Calc. phos. for malabsorption and pancreatic problems; Calc. sulph. for gushing diarrhoea; Ferr. phos. for sudden diarrhoea in a young dog; Kali mur. for pale, loose stools; Kali phos. for 'nervous' diarrhoea in a stressed dog; Nat. mur. for diarrhoea that alternates with constipation; Nat. phos. for sour, green diarrhoea; and Nat. sulph. for dark and runny stools.

Chinese medicine

The following are suggested: ground ginger (1 tsp twice daily for one week); crabapple or guava (1–3 tsps daily for one week); ginseng (50 mg tablets, or ¼ tsp of diced root, daily for one week).

supplements

Live yoghurt will help to repopulate the bowel with beneficial bacteria: 5 ml (1 tsp) should be given with each meal for one week.

urinary system

The bladder and kidneys, and their connections, form the urinary system. Symptoms of bladder problems are usually very obvious, but signs of kidney disease may be more difficult to differentiate from those of other conditions such as diabetes mellitus (see pages 80–1) or pyometra (see page 107).

Normally the first signs are seen as a change in the urine itself. This may be in the volume of urine passed, the frequency of passing urine, its colour, the presence of blood and so on. If you suspect urinary problems, it is a good idea to take a fresh sample of urine – collected in a sterile container – when you take your dog to the vet.

cystitis
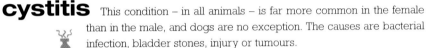
This condition – in all animals – is far more common in the female than in the male, and dogs are no exception. The causes are bacterial infection, bladder stones, injury or tumours.

Cystitis often becomes a recurrent condition, and so may require the frequent use of conventional drugs. However, the fact that natural medicines are often very effective in combating cystitis means that this reliance on conventional drugs can often be avoided. The use of natural remedies can also often help to prevent the condition from becoming a recurrent one.

Signs and symptoms Straining to pass urine very frequently, and the presence of blood in the urine.

aromatherapy
Juniper, Sandalwood and Ylang ylang may all be used for massage.

homoeopathy
Cantharis (acute dosage) is suitable for acute cystitis; Causticum, Thlaspi bursa and Equisetum (all in chronic dosage) are helpful for persistent or chronic cystitis. Vitamin C, given at a daily dosage rate of 250 mg, is another good remedy.

herbal medicine
Buchu, Couchgrass, Dandelion, Parsley, Watercress, Bearberry and Horsetail may be used as infusions.

Bach flowers
Rescue Remedy will help to relieve the discomfort of acute cystitis.

minor therapies
biochemical tissue salts
Ferr. phos. (acute dosage for three days) should be followed by Mag. phos. (chronic dosage) until the symptoms subside completely.
Chinese medicine
Hops are a good remedy: 1–3 tsps (depending on the size of the dog) should be diced into food daily.
crystals and gems
Pearl (liquid-gem remedy) may be given by mouth or added to water.

kidney disease

There are many forms of kidney disease, ranging from acute, life-threatening kidney infections to the 'wearing out' of the kidneys in old age. In addition to ageing, causes include bacterial or viral infections, poisoning and tumours.

Signs and symptoms Increased thirst, weight loss and lack of appetite; acute kidney disease may also result in vomiting, dehydration and oedema (see page 77).

aromatherapy
Juniper may be used for massage.

Bach flowers
Olive will help to alleviate weakness.

homoeopathy
Phosphorus (in acute dosage) is beneficial for acute kidney disease. Merc. sol. is suitable for a chronic condition with mouth ulcers, a wet mouth and increased thirst; Nat. mur. for increased thirst and poor skin condition (both remedies to be given in chronic dosage).

herbal medicine
Alfalfa, Cornsilk, Cleavers, Parsley and Parsnip may be given as infusions.

minor therapies
biochemical tissue salts
Ferr. phos. is suitable for an acute kidney infection; Kali phos. for a chronic kidney infection (both in acute dosage).

Chinese medicine
Root ginger and watermelon peel are both recommended: 1–3 tsps of either (depending on the size of dog), diced, should be given daily.

crystals and gems
Diamond (liquid remedy) may help.

urolithiasis

'Stones' may form in the bladder, and are occasionally found in the kidneys or urethra. They consist of minerals, including phosphate, oxalate, cystine and urate. Some are smooth, others are spiky and cause intense discomfort. The cause may be an imbalance in body fluids due to urine alkalinity or to insufficient water intake.

Signs and symptoms Blood in the urine, abdominal pain and incontinence (see opposite).

aromatherapy
Juniper may be used for massage.

homoeopathy
The following may be beneficial in a case of urolithiasis (all to be given in chronic dosage): Calc. carb. for an dog who is also overweight; Calc. phos. for a lighter and more active dog; Thlaspi bursa where phosphate stones are present; and Benzoic acid for urate stones.

 herbal medicine

Birch leaves, Couchgrass, Bearberry root and Sarsaparilla root may all be given as infusions.

minor therapies

biochemical tissue salts

Mag. phos. may be alternated with Calc. phos., or Nat. sulph. may be given (all in chronic dosage).

Chinese medicine

Star fruit is recommended: up to two fruits may be added to food daily.

crystals and gems

Pearl (liquid-gem remedy) may be given by mouth or added to water.

incontinence

 A dog who who dribbles urine is not the ideal companion, and control of incontinence is also important for the dog's comfort and health. This condition affects some neutered bitches, or may arise as part of the ageing process. Other causes are anatomical abnormalities, cystitis, and bladder 'stones' or tumours.

Signs and symptoms The urine leakage may be occasional, frequent, or almost continuous in a severe case.

Causticum cures incontinence

Charmaine was a pug with personality. She was bright, breezy and chatty (in a snuffling sort of way). And to counter the claim that dogs do not experience human emotions, I would maintain that Charmaine's embarrassment at becoming incontinent was plain for all to see.

It started with the odd dribble at night, progressed to damp patches every time she lay down, and ended as an almost continuous drip behind her. An in-depth investigation revealed no infection or other abnormality – Charmaine was simply an incontinent old lady.

Causticum – the homoeopathic remedy for problems of old age, such as stiffness and incontinence – came to the rescue. This was given twice daily for three weeks, then once daily for three further weeks. The dose is now maintained at one tablet three times a week, and Charmaine is virtually dry once again.

homoeopathy

Agnus castus is beneficial for an old male dog, and Baryta carb. for a very young or older dog of either sex (both in chronic dosage). Causticum will help to strengthen weak bladder muscles. Oestrogen is suitable for a bitch who has become incontinent since being neutered.

minor therapies

biochemical tissue salts

Calc. phos. (chronic dosage) is recommended for incontinence in an old dog.

Chinese medicine

Chestnuts or liquorice (1–3 tsps, chopped), or cinnamon (powdered, 1–3 tsps) should be given daily.

crystals and gems

Pearl (liquid-gem remedy) may be given by mouth or added to water.

female reproductive system

It seems to be the lot of the female of most species to suffer from more problems and diseases of the reproductive system than the male, and dogs are no exception to this rule. Many of these conditions are associated with pregnancy and birth.

false pregnancy

In a false pregnancy some or all of the symptoms of real pregnancy can occur, with one exception – foetuses! The cause is probably a hormonal imbalance.

Signs and symptoms Increased appetite and an enlarged abdomen, and the presence of milk in the mammary glands. The bitch may whine and refuse to settle, and, later on, may make a 'nest' and even go through mock labour 'pains'.

homoeopathy

Sepia alternated with Pulsatilla (chronic dosage) will relieve the symptoms; Cyclamen (acute dosage) helps to reduce milk secretion.

Bach flowers

Walnut will calm an anxious bitch.

minor therapies

biochemical tissue salts

Kali mur. (chronic dosage) will help many of the symptoms.

Chinese medicine

Malt reduces milk secretion: 1–3 tsps (depending on the dog's size) should be added to food daily for five days.

abortion

This is the premature expulsion of foetuses from a bitch's body before they are due to be born. Some bitches suffer from repeated abortions. The causes are various, including infection, injury, hormonal imbalance or a nutritionally poor diet.

Signs and symptoms Vaginal discharge, ejection of the dead foetuses, and general dullness, depression and lethargy.

homoeopathy

Viburnum opulis for the first three weeks; Caulophyllum for the last six weeks of pregnancy (chronic dosage).

Bach flowers

Wild rose may prevent abortion.

minor therapies

biochemical tissue salts

Calc. phos. is recommended (chronic dosage throughout pregnancy).

Chinese medicine

One to three egg yolks should be fed twice weekly throughout pregnancy.

mastitis

Inflamed mammary glands are very uncomfortable. They can also be accompanied by a high fever, bringing a risk of major damage to the glands. The cause is usually bacterial infection (especially after pregnancy or false pregnancy) or a mammary tumour.

Signs and symptoms Affected glands are hot, swollen and painful; abscesses may also form.

homoeopathy

The following are all recommended remedies for mastitis (acute dosage): Belladonna for hot, painful glands and fever; Bryonia for hot, hard glands in a dog who is unwilling to move; and Phytolacca for nodular glands.

minor therapies

biochemical tissue salts

Ferr. phos. (acute dosage) will help to alleviate the symptoms at an early stage of mastitis. Silicea (chronic dosage) should be given at a later stage, if the glands have become thickened and hardened.

Chinese medicine

A mixture of malt and crushed onion will be soothing if applied directly to the dog's mammary glands. radish leaf (chopped) or malt (1–3 tsps of either daily, depending on the size of the dog) may also be effective when added to food.

metritis and pyometra

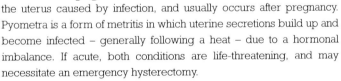

Metritis is an inflammation of the uterus caused by infection, and usually occurs after pregnancy. Pyometra is a form of metritis in which uterine secretions build up and become infected – generally following a heat – due to a hormonal imbalance. If acute, both conditions are life-threatening, and may necessitate an emergency hysterectomy.

Signs and symptoms Vaginal discharge, fever, increased thirst and loss of appetite.

aromatherapy

Sage may be used for massage.

homoeopathy

The following are beneficial (all given in acute dosage unless specified): Caulophyllum for chocolate-coloured vaginal discharge; Helonias for hindquarter weakness; Hydrastis in early pyometra with a large amount of catarrhal discharge; Sabina when copious fresh blood is present in the discharge; and Sepia for persistent chronic metritis or pyometra (chronic dosage).

herbal medicine

Goldenseal, Myrrh and Rose hips may all be given by infusion and will help to relieve the symptoms.

eclampsia

Also commonly known as milk fever, eclampsia is more likely to affect a bitch who has a large litter. It is a tetanus-like condition (see page 119) that can occur while the bitch is feeding her puppies. The cause is a calcium and/or glucose deficiency.

Signs and symptoms Restlessness, a high fever, panting, muscle tremors and convulsions.

homoeopathy
Belladonna (acute dosage) will be helpful; this should be followed by Calc. phos. (chronic dosage).

minor therapies
biochemical tissue salts
Ferr. phos. (acute dosage) should be given initially for three days. This should be followed by Mag. phos. alternated with Calc. phos. (both to be given in chronic dosage).

crystals and gems
Diamond (liquid-gem remedy) can be effective: this may be given by mouth or added to drinking water.

infertility

In many instances, no specific cause can be found for a lack of fertility in a bitch – it could simply result from an unsuccessful mating. Alternatively, the problem may be due to a combination of factors such as stress, obesity, hormonal imbalance, abnormalities of the reproductive organs and infections, or, of course, to problems with the stud dog.

Signs and symptoms A bitch with fertility problems will either not become pregnant, or will only produce small litters.

homoeopathy
Sepia should be given alternately with Pulsatilla (chronic dosage). Platina (chronic dosage) may also be helpful.

herbal medicine
Raspberry leaf should be given as an infusion.

Bach flowers
Clematis is indicated when there is a lack of interest by the bitch; Larch will help where there is a lack of self-confidence or shyness.

minor therapies
biochemical tissue salts
Nat. mur. (chronic dosage) is an effective remedy.

Chinese medicines
Ginseng may be given at a dose rate of 10–30 mg daily, or fresh shrimps at the rate of 25–75 g (1–3 oz) daily.

supplements
A course of royal jelly is a general health supplement to keep a bitch in peak condition. Fresh (not the freeze-dried version) of royal jelly should always be given if available.

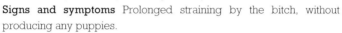

dystocia
Difficulty in giving birth is less common in dogs than in humans, mainly because bitches usually have several small babies, rather than one large one. Where problems do arise, the cause may be a hormonal imbalance, stress, or abnormal foetuses. Natural medicines are extremely useful in promoting an easy birth.

Signs and symptoms Prolonged straining by the bitch, without producing any puppies.

aromatherapy
Lavender and Sage are both helpful when used for gentle massage several days before the birth.

homoeopathy
Caulophyllum may be given during pregnancy (chronic dosage) and birth (acute dosage). Given immediately after the birth, Arnica (acute dosage) will reduce bruising around the vulva.

herbal medicine
Infusions of Raspberry leaf given throughout pregnancy will help to prevent problems with the birth.

Bach flowers
Walnut may be given during the pregnancy. At the time of labour, oak will help a bitch who has stopped straining to 'try harder'; Star of Bethlehem will encourage a bitch to resume straining if she has stopped in fear or panic.

minor therapies
biochemical tissue salts
Calc. fluor. should be alternated with Kali phos. (acute dosage).

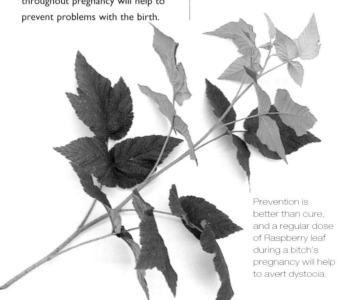

Prevention is better than cure, and a regular dose of Raspberry leaf during a bitch's pregnancy will help to avert dystocia.

agalactia

This condition arises when a new mother has inadequate milk. Either a little milk or no milk at all may be produced as a result of a hormonal imbalance, stress or mastitis (see page 107).

Signs and symptoms A litter of hungry puppies usually reveals agalactia very rapidly!

homoeopathy
Calc. phos. or Lecithin (both in acute dosage) may be beneficial.

herbal medicine
Milk wort, Milk thistle, Goat's rue, Marshmallow and Fennel all have a milk-producing capacity.

aiding milk production

There was no mistaking the fact that Jenny, a young Irish setter, was having problems in coping with her new role in life. To become a mother at two years of age must be quite an experience – especially to a litter of seven noisy puppies.

Jenny seemed to try hard: she barely rested and was always checking, cleaning and feeding her offspring. Perhaps the responsibility had become too much, but something caused her supply of milk to dry up. The more the puppies cried, the less milk she produced.

A herbalist friend supplied Milkwort, and I recommended that this should be made into an infusion and administered twice daily. I supplied homoeopathic Calc. phos. (to be given in acute dosage). The owners created as soothing and calming an atmosphere as was possible, with plenty of attention and support for Jenny, and plenty of food and fluids. The milk returned very rapidly, and within four days the puppies were well-fed and contented again.

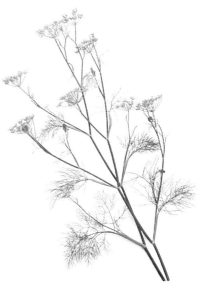

Fennel is one of several herbs that have a natural ability to stimulate milk production.

Bach flowers
Crabapple acts as a cleansing remedy.

minor therapies
biochemical tissue salts
Kali mur. (acute dosage) will help.
Chinese medicine
The following will encourage milk: dill seed, asparagus, lettuce seed, sesame seed, chicken with ginger and dried shrimp (1–3 tsps daily, depending on dog's size).
crystals and gems
Ruby (liquid-gem remedy) may be given by mouth or added to water.

male reproductive system

Male dogs may not suffer from the same variety of problems affecting the reproductive system that bitches do, but they still have their own small range of conditions that affect the testicles, prostate gland and penis.

prostatitis

Inflammation of the prostate gland may be a chronic enlargement that occurs as part of ageing and places pressure on the bowels and/or the bladder; or an acute problem, usually following infection tracking up from the urethra. Tumours are another cause.

Signs and symptoms Pain, difficulty in passing urine and faeces, and the presence of blood in the urine.

homoeopathy

Clematis is suitable for a young dog who is experiencing difficulty in passing urine; and Ipecac. should be administered when there is a considerable quantity of blood in the urine (both in acute dosage). The following are also beneficial (all in chronic dosage): Sabal serrulata for a young or old dog who is suffering from chronic prostatitis; Agnus castus for an older dog who has an enlarged prostate gland and shrunken testicles; and Nux vomica when the dog is having difficulty in passing faeces.

minor therapies

biochemical tissue salts
Silica (chronic dosage) is a very good remedy in a case of chronic prostate enlargement.
Chinese medicine
Cottonseed may be administered as an infusion.

a gentle cure – Sabal serrulata

Lloyd was a lovely old German shepherd dog, greying and starting to slow down, but still a fine figure of a dog. Like many older males – human or canine – he was beginning to suffer from prostate problems and had difficulty in emptying his bowels and in passing urine (the latter often including traces of blood).

I chose homoeopathic Sabal serrulata to begin treatment, to be given at the chronic dosage for two weeks. Lloyd's owner was very anxious that this therapy should work, as the conventional approach to prostate problems is castration which, in a dog of Lloyd's age (about 12) would have involved some degree of anaesthetic risk.

The treatment was successful and, after three weeks, Lloyd was more comfortable. The remedy was reduced to once daily for two weeks, then to once twice weekly. On this 'maintenance' dose Lloyd – although he still has a slightly enlarged prostate – has virtually no symptoms, and is growing old gracefully.

hypersexuality

The only complete cure for uncontrollable hypersexuality in a male dog may be castration, although many young dogs do 'grow out' of this behaviour and castration is not the answer in every case. Hypersexual behaviour is often due to a hormonal imbalance, but it can also result from habitual learned behaviour – just as children learn and continue bad habits, so can dogs.

Signs and symptoms Aggression, roaming, mounting animate and inanimate objects and destructive behaviour.

aromatherapy
Lavender and Sweet marjoram essential oils, used for massage, will have a calming influence.

homoeopathy
The following are good remedies (all in chronic dosage): Cantharis, especially if the hypersexuality is accompanied by an irritable bladder; phosphorus for a nervous, excitable dog; Tarentula hisp. for a hysterical dog who may be snappy; and Ustillago maydis for a dog who has swollen testicles and is very active sexually.

herbal medicine
Skullcap with Valerian, or Hops, may both be given by infusion (Skullcap with Valerian is also available in the form of proprietary tablets).

Bach flowers
Vervain is a suitable remedy for an 'over-enthusiastic' dog; Impatiens for an irritable and excitable one.

minor therapies
biochemical tissue salts
Mag. phos. (chronic dosage) may be beneficial.

orchitis

Orchitis is inflammation of the testicles, and is one of the most painful conditions to affect male dogs. This disorder may be caused by injury, bacterial infection or a tumour.

Signs and symptoms Painful, swollen testicles. The pain could grow so acute that the dog stops eating, and passing urine may be difficult.

homoeopathy
Belladonna (acute dosage) is beneficial. Also suitable at a later stage, for hardened testicles, are Bryonia (acute dosage), especially where there is pressure; and Rhododendron, where the testicles are scarred (chronic dosage).

minor therapies
biochemical tissue salts
Ferr. phos. (acute dosage) will help to relieve the swelling.
Chinese medicine
Kelp powder is advised: 1–2 tsps (depending on the size of the dog) should be added to food daily.

cancer

Cancerous tissue can grow in any part of any body organ. Some tumours – such as skin tumours – are obvious, but others may go unnoticed until they are quite advanced. Cancer seems to be increasing in incidence in dogs, perhaps because they are living longer. Some forms of the disease – such as bone cancer (osteosarcoma), mast-cell tumours and melanomas (forms of skin cancer), and lymphoma (lymph-gland cancer) – are surprisingly common in fairly young dogs. Natural remedies can contain and even cure cancer, and will certainly help to relieve symptoms even in a terminal case.

One possible reason for the upsurge of cancer cases in dogs may be the amount of pollutants in the environment, which damage the immune system and reduce the natural ability of the body to destroy cancer cells at an early stage. Supplements to keep dogs at peak health and fitness (see pages 46–8) are therefore very important.

aromatherapy
Rosemary and Ylang ylang, used for massage, will be revitalizing for an old dog afflicted with cancer.

homoeopathy
Hydrastis will help in an early case of cancer, while Arsen. alb. relieves pain and suffering in terminal cancer (both in acute dosage). Echinacea (chronic dosage) helps the immune system to fight cancer. Viscum alb. (chronic dosage) – the homoeopathic remedy made from mistletoe – is also beneficial in most cases.

herbal medicine
Good results have been achieved by giving Mistletoe extract by injection. Infusions of Echinacea tincture, Red clover and Autumn crocus may also be used. Apricot kernels, ground and kept cool, and given at a dosage rate of 25–75 mg (depending on the size of dog) twice daily, have been shown to be beneficial in cancer cases (note that the kernels must not be kept in water, as this can cause a reaction that will liberate a toxin).

Bach flowers
Crabapple is an excellent general cleansing remedy. Other effective treatments include Hornbeam, to give strength to a weakened dog; Mimulus for one who seems to be frightened by his or her symptoms; and Olive to aid a dog who appears to have lost the will to live.

minor therapies
biochemical tissue salts
Calc. phos. (chronic dosage) helps to tone the metabolism.
Chinese medicine
Job's tears and shiitake mushrooms are the recommended Chinese remedies for cancer: 2–6 tsps of each food, finely chopped, should be given daily. Beetroot juice is also suitable: 5–15 ml (1–3 tsps) should be administered daily.

supplements
The following vitamins will help to strengthen the immune system, and to detoxify poisons produced by cancerous tissue (the amounts indicated are daily doses, and vary according to the size of the dog): Vitamin A (1000–3000 iu); B-complex vitamins – in the form of Brewer's yeast – (3–6 tsps); Vitamin C (2–6 g); and Vitamin E (200–600 iu). Garlic, royal jelly and aloe vera added to the diet will also help to stabilize metabolic processes in the body.

therapies give longer life

Peter was a retired racing greyhound. Dogs of this type make wonderful pets – quiet, loving, and needing very little in life. Peter had recently become lame in his right foreleg, with a swelling appearing at the shoulder joint. X-rays had revealed that a bone tumour (osteosarcoma) was developing. This is a malignant tumour, usually rapidly growing, and capable of spreading to the lungs and sometimes to other parts of the body. It can also cause considerable pain and lameness. Determined to do everything possible for Peter, his owner brought him to me for natural therapy.

I began a course of acupuncture, using points such as large intestine 15 (Jianyu) and Gall bladder 21 (Jianjing), which help to relieve pain and to encourage healing. The acupuncture sessions were given twice weekly for the first four weeks. I also prescribed the homoeopathic remedies Hydrastis and Viscum alb. (to be given in chronic dosage), both of which are anti-cancer remedies. Finally, I added the Bach flower essences of Hornbeam (strengthening) and Olive (for loss of willpower – Peter seemed very depressed), with one drop of each to be given twice daily.

During the first four weeks, the swelling did not increase in size, and Peter did not deteriorate in general condition. I reduced the acupuncture to once weekly for a further four weeks, then to once every two weeks. The homoeopathic dosage was reduced to once daily for two weeks, then to one dose twice weekly. During this time Peter's condition remained stable, and he remained well for several months, with just a slight lameness and no pain.

Eventually the tumour did become active again, and Peter's life finally had to be brought to an end. However, his period of remission gave him many extra months of happy, active life that without the natural medicines would not have been possible.

parasites

A good natural diet and a healthy lifestyle should ensure that parasites are kept to a minimum, but even healthy dogs will occasionally be host to internal parasites such as roundworms and tapeworms, and to a number of external parasites. Natural therapies can play an important role in preventing parasites and resolving an infestation.

surface-dwelling parasites

Fleas, lice, ticks, cheyletiella ('rabbit-fur' mites) and harvest mites live on the skin's surface, and can all affect dogs. Fleas are dark brown insects that run rapidly through the fur. Lice are slow-moving grey insects and are often found in clusters, particularly on the ear flaps. Ticks resemble smooth, grey warts; they fix their mouth parts into the skin and do not move. Cheyletiella often affect puppies of short-coated breeds (an infestation is sometimes called 'walking dandruff'), while orange harvest mites affect the feet, legs and stomach areas.

Signs and symptoms In addition to visible signs, the dog may scratch and groom excessively to relieve the irritation caused by fleas, lice or mites. There could also be a bumpy, allergic reaction to the bites.

aromatherapy

Cedarwood, Eucalyptus, Terebinth, Lemon, Rosemary, Lavender and Mint may be used for massage, or diluted and brushed into the fur (see right).

(5 ml [1 tsp] per 600 ml [1 pt] of drinking water) is a good preventive measure; alternatively, a dog may be bathed daily in a solution of ⅓ vinegar to ⅔ water, for fleas.

Cedarwood, Eucalyptus, Terebinth, Mint, Lemon, Lavender and Rosemary all help to prevent surface-dwelling parasites. Any of these oils may be used for massage, or can be added to water (three drops per 150 ml [¼ pt] water) and then combed or brushed into the dog's fur.

homoeopathy

One tablet of Sulphur should be given weekly to prevent fleas. Pulex (chronic dosage) soothes irritation.

herbal medicine

Pennyroyal, Tansy and Fleabane are flea-repelling: they can be sprinkled on carpets and the dog's bedding.

minor therapies

supplements

Brewer's yeast may be given orally, or combed into the fur. Cider vinegar

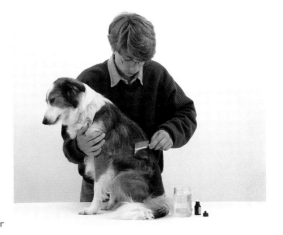

burrowing mites

Also called mange mites, there are two species of burrowing mites that affect dogs: sarcoptes and demodex. They are more difficult to eradicate than surface-dwelling parasites. Demodectic mange usually occurs if there is an immune-system deficiency, and is notoriously hard to eliminate.

Signs and symptoms Excessive scratching, resulting in reddened skin and alopecia (see pages 62–3).

aromatherapy
Lemon, Lavender and Wild marjoram may be used for massage, or diluted (three drops per 150 ml [¼ pt] of water) and then brushed into the fur.

homoeopathy
Sulphur is beneficial for a dog with mange who avoids heat; Psorinum for a dog who seeks heat.

herbal medicine
Lemon and Pomegranate juice (5 ml [1 tsp] of each per 300 ml [½ pt] water) may be used to wash the skin. Garlic (⅓ to one chopped clove, depending on the size of dog) should be added to food daily.

minor therapies
biochemical tissue salts
Calc. sulph. (chronic dosage) will help to eliminate burrowing mites.
Chinese medicine
Sesame oil is the recommended remedy: 2.5–10 ml (½–2 tsps), depending on the size of dog, should be added to the diet daily.
crystals and gems
Sapphire (liquid remedy) may help.

ear mites

These creatures – known as otodectic mites – live inside a dog's ears. They can cause intense irritation and lead to conditions such as aural haematoma and otitis media (see pages 67 and 68), but the following natural medicines will all help.

Signs and symptoms Excessive scratching of the ears, head-shaking, and a black discharge coming from the ears.

homoeopathy
Sulphur is beneficial for a dog with ear mites who avoids heat; Psorinum for one who seeks heat.

herbal medicine
Olive oil (15 ml [3 tsps]) and Vitamin E (500 iu) should be mixed and used to clean the ears twice daily. Thyme, Rosemary, Rue and Teatree may all be given by mouth, or used to clean the outer part of the ears. Calendula lotion can also be used to clean the ears, and is very soothing for sore, reddened areas caused by scratching.

ringworm

Ringworm (dermatophytosis) is a fungal skin infection that is generally passed on by direct contact between dogs.

Signs and symptoms In most cases – but not always – circular patches of hair loss occur, and the affected skin is itchy and sore.

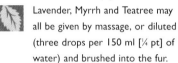

aromatherapy

Lavender, Myrrh and Teatree may all be given by massage, or diluted (three drops per 150 ml [¼ pt] of water) and brushed into the fur.

homoeopathy

Bacillinum, Tellurium, Sepia and Kali arsen. (chronic dosage) are helpful.

herbal medicine

Goldenseal or Echinacea tincture should be applied to affected areas of the skin daily.

minor therapies

crystals and gems

Sapphire (liquid-gem remedy) may be given by mouth or added to water.

worms

Parasitic worms in the intestinal tract are all too common, especially in puppies. Tapeworms are carried by fleas, so flea-infested dogs will be most at risk. Other worms found in dogs include hookworms, whipworms and – very rarely in the UK – heartworms, which live in a dog's arteries.

Signs and symptoms Roundworms and tapeworms may be visible in the faeces. Roundworms are thin, white, round-bodied and up to 15 cm (6 in) long; tapeworms appear as flat, short segments resembling large grains of rice (the main tapeworm remains in the intestine) and may be found around the anus or on a dog's bedding.

aromatherapy

Bergamot, Thyme and Marjoram may all be used for massage.

homoeopathy

Cina or Chenopodium is effective for roundworms; Granatum or Filix mas for tapeworms. One dose should be given twice daily for three days, every four weeks, as a preventive measure.

herbal medicine

Rue may be given as an infusion.

minor therapies

biochemical tissue salts

Nat. phos. (chronic dosage) is a helpful remedy for worms.

Chinese medicine

Papaya (chopped) and coconut (grated) are advised: 1–3 tsps of each (depending on the size of the dog) should be given. In addition, 2–6 tsps of carrot (grated), pumpkin seeds (ground), pomegranate rind (powdered) or melon pips may be added to the dog's food daily.

specific infections

All dogs are at risk of contracting a variety of infectious diseases, although the lifestyle of an individual will obviously influence the likelihood of picking up an infection (vaccinations are available for some of these diseases: consult your vet for further advice). The most important diseases to affect dogs are included here. The specific symptoms that they produce (such as coughing, vomiting, and so on) can be treated with reference to appropriate sections of the book. All the diseases listed will also benefit from the treatments outlined on the opposite page.

canine parvovirus

A viral infection, this disease affects both the digestive system and the heart, causing severe vomiting and diarrhoea with blood. In young puppies, it may also result in heart damage.

distemper

Distemper is a viral infection that affects many parts of the body. The symptoms include fever, coughing, nasal discharge, conjunctivitis, diarrhoea, and convulsions (fits) or chorea.

canine hepatitis

This viral infection attacks a dog's liver, causing vomiting, diarrhoea, fever, abdominal pain and sometimes jaundice.

canine leptospirosis

There are two forms of this bacterial infection. One form affects the liver and causes jaundice, diarrhoea and vomiting; the other causes kidney damage, and produces accompanying symptoms of mouth ulcers, excessive thirst and vomiting.

'kennel cough'

A combination of a viral and bacterial infection, kennel cough is prevalent in situations where there are many dogs – such as at boarding kennels or dog shows – enabling the rapid transmission of the disease. It affects the respiratory system, resulting in a sore throat and persistent coughing.

lyme disease

This is a bacterial disease spread by ticks. This mainly affects the musculo-skeletal system, resulting in obvious lameness, but it can also cause heart damage.

aspergillosis

This is a fungal infecton affecting the respiratory system. It causes nasal discharge, coughing and sometimes epistaxis (nose bleeds).

neosporosis

This is a protozoal disease that affects the musculo-skeletal system, causing paralysis and stiffness of the legs (usually the hindlegs).

tetanus

Tetanus is a bacterial infection that affects the nervous system. It causes muscle stiffness and paralysis, especially of the jaw.

toxoplasmosis

This is another protozoal infection. It affects various parts of the body and produces a number of different symptoms, including weight loss, coughing, nasal discharge, diarrhoea and abortions in bitches.

The following therapies will be beneficial for all specific infections.

aromatherapy

Lemon combined with Sage may be massaged into the skin.

homoeopathy

Aconite should be given at the earliest sign of disease; Belladonna when there is a high fever and the symptoms are severe (both in acute dosage). Specific nosodes to most diseases are also available (for example, Distemper nosode and Kennel-cough nosode). There is also some evidence that a nosode will help to prevent the occurrence of a particular disease.

herbal medicine

Goldenseal and Echinacea may both be used as tinctures. Garlic is a good general preventive remedy: ⅓ to one chopped clove (depending on the size of the dog) should be added to food daily.

Bach flowers

Rescue Remedy is beneficial for any disease whose symptoms are acute.

minor therapies

biochemical tissue salts

Ferr. phos. (acute dosage) will be helpful to relieve acute symptoms.

crystals and gems

Pearl (liquid-gem remedy) may be given by mouth or added to water.

supplements

Given as a dietary supplement, Vitamin C will help the body to fight specific diseases. At times of acute infection, 1–3 g (depending on the size of the dog) should be given daily.

behaviour

Behavioural problems in dogs seem to be on the increase, and many dogs exhibit the same kinds of anxieties or hyperactivity seen in some children and adults. To help prevent the development of such problems, the following factors must be borne in mind.

• Only go to see a litter whose parents you know to be calm and well-behaved. Choose a puppy who is neither shy and withdrawn when handled, nor too bouncy and boisterous.

• One common reason for problems of fear and aggression in young dogs is lack of proper socialization: between six and 12 weeks of age, puppies must be introduced to dogs and humans of all shapes and sizes, and learn how to react normally to them.

• Train your puppy: dog-training classes are helpful, but training must also be carried through to everyday activities. Do not let your puppy become dominant in the home – allowing him or her to sleep in your bed, to sit on chairs, to eat before you do or to pull on the lead while out on walks will all cause problems later.

• A good, well-balanced diet will help to produce a good, well-balanced dog. Vitamin deficiencies, protein excess and mineral imbalance can all lead to or aggravate behaviour problems.

If behaviour problems have developed, seek advice quickly. Trained behaviour counsellors (your vet will refer you if necessary) employ a range of techniques, gradually reinforcing good behaviour in the dog while discouraging unwanted behaviour. However, some problems are unresponsive to training methods or behavioural therapy, and this is where natural medicines can come into their own: for instance, many persistent behavioural disorders in dogs respond rapidly to a course of acupuncture or to T-touch massage.

Choosing the right puppy is a vital first step in ensuring that behavioural problems do not arise later on. A puppy who is friendly and playful but not over-boisterous, nor very timid and withdrawn, will make the ideal pet for most families.

nervousness

Accidents, physical or mental abuse by humans, or even undergoing a routine vaccination can lead to anxiety. Some dogs are frightened of thunderstorms; some are scared of other dogs or vacuum cleaners. Such anxieties can affect dogs at different levels. Some experience a mild nervous reaction to certain stimuli; others are constantly 'highly strung'. Some dogs are fairly calm generally, but exhibit an almost phobic reaction in specific situations. Events such as being attacked by another animal can spark nervousness, although some dogs appear to be born this way, which is a good reason for choosing a puppy carefully (see opposite).

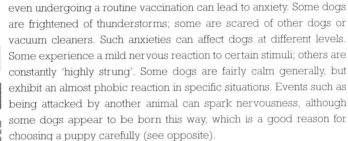

aromatherapy
Massage with Camomile, Lavender, Lemon balm, Neroli or Sweet marjoram will have a calming effect.

homoeopathy
The following are effective remedies (all given in chronic dosage): Aconite for nervousness that begins after a frightening experience; Argent. nit. for the 'hurried and worried' dog; Gelsemium for a dog who becomes almost rigid with fear (this is often used for stagefright in humans); and Phosphorus, especially for fear of sudden noises.

herbal remedies
A range of infusions will be very beneficial. Camomile is soothing, as is common oat. Hops given as a herbal infusion are extremely helpful for a neurotic dog, while Passiflora will pacify and soothe an anxious one. An infusion of Vervain is another good choice for lack of confidence. Skullcap with Valerian – available as proprietary tablets – makes a classic herbal calming remedy.

Bach flowers
Aspen is ideal for general background anxiety; Mimulus for fear of specific situations; and Rock rose for severe phobias and panic attacks.

acupuncture
This is a very useful therapy for a nervous dog.

minor therapies
biochemical tissue salts
Mag. phos. (chronic dosage) is an excellent 'nerve tonic'.
Chinese medicine
Oystershell may be given, as a few fragments crumbled with each meal. Dates or longans (1 tsp) with food every two to three days helps to calm a nervous disposition. A few petals of lily flower – known in Chinese medicine as the sorrow-forgetting flower – added to food every few days is helpful for the 'worried' dog.
crystals and gems
Pearl (liquid-gem remedy) is very 'nourishing' for the nervous system and will help to calm a fractious dog.

aggression

Aggression is a natural instinct that is useful when a dog is guarding a house or his owners, but it must always be controllable. Where a dog has a tendency to be over-aggressive, the following remedies will be beneficial.

aromatherapy

Sandalwood and Ylang ylang may be used for massage, or administered via a diffuser.

homoeopathy

The following are effective remedies (all to be administered in chronic dosage): Belladonna for anger and a tendency to bite; Nux vomica for irritability; Staphisagria for apparent feelings of resentment; Lachesis for jealousy of any kind; and Hyoscyamus for feelings of rage.

herbal medicine

Camomile, given as an infusion, has a wonderfully soothing effect on an aggressive dog. Skullcap with Valerian (available combined, in the form of proprietary tablets) is also good for calming aggressive behaviour.

Bach flowers

Holly is ideal for rage and general aggression; Impatiens for irritability and a tendency towards snappiness; and Willow for feelings of anger and resentment.

acupuncture

As is the case with many behavioural problems, a course of this treatment is often rapidly effective at resolving aggressive behaviour.

reducing aggression

I have known some aggressive dogs in my time – all proponents of the 'bite first, ask questions later' policy – but Hogan was one of the worst. Just a look in his direction and a snarl would erupt. Dare to approach him, and a warning growl through bared teeth would be heard. Try to examine him, and you would never play the piano again. I think I was more scared of Hogan than any of my other patients – and, embarrassingly, he is a chihuahua.

I wish – wholeheartedly – that natural remedies had turned Hogan into a sweet, loving dog. They have not done so, but they have helped, with the counsel of a behaviour therapist, to make him a more approachable and better-natured animal. I advised the Bach flowers Holly (for rage and aggression) and Impatiens (for irritability): one drop twice daily for four weeks, then one drop twice weekly. I also prescribed the herbal calming remedy Skullcap with Valerian (one tablet daily). However, I did not try to give the tablets myself!

minor therapies

T-touch massage

This treatment can be very beneficial for instilling a sense of calm, and for soothing fractiousness.

crystals and gems

Pearl or Onyx (liquid-gem remedy) may be given by mouth or added to drinking water.

hyperactivity

Certain breeds of dog – such as the Irish setter, boxer, border collie and dalmatian – are simply born with a great deal of energy. In these breeds in particular there appears to be a predisposition to hyperactivity, but a dog of any breed can be prone to excess energy. However, a distinction must be drawn between normal high spirits and true hyperactivity, in which persistent wakefulness, repetitive behaviour and manic activity are evident.

Hyperactivity can sometimes be linked to food additives, and there is also some evidence that very high levels of protein in the diet can be a factor, so these should be avoided (your vet will give you advice on feeding the optimum diet for a hyperactive dog). In many instances there is no known reason for the condition, and it is here that natural therapies can be of great benefit.

aromatherapy

Lavender, Sweet marjoram and Camomile essential oils may all be used for massage: not only the oils, but also the massage itself can have a very relaxing effect.

homoeopathy

The following will be beneficial (all to be administered in chronic dosage): Belladonna for an excitable and aggressive dog; Coffea for sleeplessness and an obvious lack of concentration; and Stramonium, Scutellaria or Tarentula for a dog with odd behaviour patterns, such as catching imaginary flies.

herbal medicine

Skullcap with Valerian may be given in tablet form, and Melissa (lemon balm) or Hops as infusions.

Bach flowers

Vervain will have a soothing effect on a hyperactive dog; White chestnut will have a calming effect on a dog who is restless at night; Heather is effective for the dog who always demands attention; and Scleranthus is useful for erratic behaviour – for example, the dog who never runs in a straight line, and who is prone to sudden changes of mood.

acupuncture

This treatment can have a very calming effect if sessions are carried out on a regular basis.

minor therapies

biochemical tissue salts

Kali phos. (chronic dosage) is often extremely helpful.

T-touch massage

A course of massage can be very effective for reducing hyperactivity and wakefulness.

crystals and gems

Sapphire (liquid-gem remedy) may be given directly by mouth or added to drinking water.

pining and grief

Dogs who are put in boarding kennels – even for relatively short periods – can seem to feel abandoned, while those moving to new homes may suffer from a form of homesickness. Dogs also grieve for members of the family, or for canine companions, and can even develop physical disease as a result. If your dog is a puppy, accustoming him or her to short periods of separation from you from an early age is a very good idea.

aromatherapy
Basil, Bergamot and Orange blossom will help a dog through a period of emotional trauma.

homoeopathy
Ignatia (given in chronic dosage) – the principal homoeopathic remedy for grief and pining – is invaluable in stressful situations. Pulsatilla (given in chronic dosage) is ideal for the shy and reserved type of dog who has become withdrawn.

herbal medicine
Lime blossom – given in the form of infusions – will assist a dog in overcoming the emotional trauma of a bereavement.

Bach flowers
Honeysuckle is helpful for pining; Walnut helps at times of transition.

minor therapies
T-touch massage
This will be beneficial in many cases.

coprophagia

The unpleasant habit of eating their own faeces is surprisingly common among dogs. Some do this occasionally, some all the time; other dogs spread their net wider and eat cat, sheep, cattle and horse droppings. It is a common misconception that dogs eat their own droppings due to vitamin or mineral deficiency, although those with digestive abnormalities may pass partially undigested food in their faeces, and retrieve this by coprophagia.

A dried-food diet should be given (this produces more compact, perhaps less edible faeces), and any droppings removed as soon as possible. The following may also help.

homoeopathy
Calc. carb. and China officinalis (both to be administered in chronic dosage) can help to resolve the habit of faeces-eating, especially if they are given at an early stage.

minor therapies
supplements
Pineapple chunks added to the diet seem to give the faeces an unpleasant taste, and therefore can act as a deterrent to many dogs.

travel sickness

True motion sickness is probably less common than anxiety and apprehension about travelling. However, many dogs suffer from one or both of these problems with travelling. Behavioural therapy can be very effective: this usually consists of gradually accustoming the dog first to being in a stationary car, then to being in the car with the engine running, then to the car being driven a short distance, and so on. Natural medicines can speed up this process, or are often effective on their own.

aromatherapy

Sweet fennel, Peppermint and Camomile, used for massage, will all help to reduce feelings of anxiety.

homoeopathy

Cocculus, Borax and Petroleum are very effective; Tabacum is particularly good for seasickness and airsickness (all remedies should be given in acute dosage before the journey).

herbal medicine

Peppermint helps to allay anxiety. Hanging bunches of Parsley in the car also mysteriously seems to prevent travel sickness in some dogs!

Bach flowers

Scleranthus is helpful in many cases.

minor therapies

biochemical tissue salts

Kali phos. (chronic dosage) will help to alleviate nausea.

supplements

B-complex vitamins can be an effective dietary supplement for a dog who is prone to travel sickness. Feeding some ginger biscuits before a journey is helpful in some cases.

using a range of therapies

Kipper was a three-year-old Scottish terrier who enjoyed everything about life – except travelling in a car. Within the first few minutes of any and every journey, he would begin to lick his lips, dribble and then to howl disconsolately. Only rarely did he actually vomit, but the feeling of nausea and misery was self-evident.

Fortunately, homoeopathic remedies were a great help. Cocculus and Petroleum (both given in acute dosage, for one hour before a journey), followed by a few drops of the Bach flower Rescue Remedy just as the journey was about to commence, improved the situation a great deal.

Prior to a longer trip of several hours, Peppermint infusion was given twice daily for three days beforehand, as well as the other homoeopathic remedies on the day of the journey. While still not exactly a seasoned traveller, Kipper is certainly now able to cope with car journeys without unduly upsetting himself – or his owners.

appendix

Some homoeopathic remedies are commonly known by abbreviations of their Latin names, and have been included in these abbreviated forms throughout this book. The abbreviations and full names of the remedies used are listed below.

Abbreviation	Full name	Abbreviation	Full name
Acid. nit.	Acidum nitricum	Hydrastis	Hydrastis canadensis
Acid. phos.	Acidum phosphoricum	Ipecac. syrup	Ipecacuanha
Acid. sal.	Acidum salicylicum	Iris vers.	Iris versicolor
Aconite	Aconitum napellus	Kali arsen.	Kali arsenicosum
Ant. crud.	Antimonium crudum	Kali bich.	Kali bichromium
Argent. nit.	Argentum nitricum	Kali carb.	Kali carbonica
Arsen. alb.	Aresenicum album	Kali chlor.	Kali chloricum
Baryta carb.	Baryta carbonica	Kali mur.	Kali muriaticum
Bryonia	Bryonia alba	Kali sulph.	Kali sulphuricum
Cactus grand.	Cactus grandiflorus	Lycopodium	Lycopodium clavatum
Calc. carb.	Calcarea carbonica	Mag. phos.	Magnesia phosphorica
Calc. fluor.	Calcarea fluorica	Merc. cor.	Mericurius corrosivus
Calc. phos.	Calcarea phosphorica	Merc. sol.	Mericurius solubilis
Carduus	Carduus marianus	Nat. mur.	Natrum muriaticum
Caulophyllum	Caulophyllum thalictroides	Plumb. met.	Plumbum metallicum
Chelidonium	Chelidonium majus	Pulsatilla	Pulsatilla nigricans
Cocculus	Cocculus indicus	Rhus tox.	Rhus toxicodendron
Colchicum	Colchicum autumnale	Ruta grav.	Ruta graveolens
Conium mac.	Conium maculatum	Tarentula hisp.	Tarentula hispanica
Cuprum met.	Cuprum metallicum	Thuja	Thuja occidentalis
Echinalea	Echinalea augustifolia	Ver. alb.	Veratrum album
Ferrum met.	Ferrum metallicum	Viscum alb.	Viscum album
Hepar sulph.	Hepar sulphuris calcareum	Zinc. met.	Zincum metallicum

acknowledgements

Reed Illustrated Books would like to thank Jane Burton (and her dogs Emma and Hamilton), Jackie Chambers, Kate Dunning, Britta Stent (and Pippa), Hazel Taylor (and Lark), Lisë Whittle (and Daisy) and Linnea Taylor for their help with photography.

ILLUSTRATIONS: Greg Poole 8-9, 50–1; Annette Whalley 26

PHOTOGRAPHS: Mary Evans Picture Library/John Cutten 21

Reed International Books Ltd/Jane Burton 1, 2–3, 10, 11, 17, 18, 19, 23 right, 23 left, 25, 29, 32, 33, 38, 39, 42, 48, 49 left, 49 right, 54 right, 54 left, 61, 64 left, 64 right, 69 left, 69 right, 80, 83, 85, 89, 93, 96, 109, 110, 115; Peter Chadwick (courtesy of Hahnemann Museum) 13; Warren Photographic/Jane Burton 120, front cover

index

abdominal pain 98, 99, 103, 104, 118
abortion 106, 118, 119
abscess 65, 94
accidents 52–9, 86
  bites and stings 55
  burns 59
  collapse 82
  and shock 57
  haemorrhaging 56
  heatstroke 59
  poisoning 58
  wounds 54–5
acupuncture 6, 7, 24–7, 84
  electro-acupuncture 25
  laser treatment 26
  meridians 24, 26
  moxibustion 25
Addison's disease 82
additives 41, 123
administering tablets 15, 49
agalactia 110
ageing 61, 64
aggression 112, 122
air 38–9
allergies 40, 60, 73
alopecia 62–3, 81, 82
anaemia 78–9
anal-gland disorders 63
anaphylactic shock 57
antibiotics 51, 72
anxiety 21, 120
appetite
  increased 80, 106
  lack of 72, 96, 100, 104, 107
aromatherapy 7, 9, 10–12, 115
arthritis 6, 10, 14, 16, 19, 24, 25, 47, 80, 83–4, 87
artificial respiration 53
ascites 77, 100
aspergillosis 74, 118
auto-immune disease 27, 78

Bach, Dr Edward 21
Bach flowers 7, 21–3
bad breath see halitosis
balance, loss of 68, 91
baldness see alopecia
bandaging 53, 86
B-complex vitamins 48
behaviour 120–5
  changes in 92
  therapy 120, 123
biochemical tissue salts 9, 28
birth 109
bites and stings 55

bladder 'stones' 103, 104, 105
bleeding 56, 75
  controlling 53, 56
blindness 71
blood clotting 56, 78
blood loss 56, 78
boarding kennels 73, 118, 124
body temperature, raised 59
bones 47; see also musculo-skeletal system
  fracture 86, 90
  new growth of 88
brain 91
  inflammation 92
  tumour 91
breathlessness 76
brucellosis 118
burns 59, 62

cancer 47, 113–14
canine hepatitis 100, 118
canine leptospirosis 118
canine parvovirus 118
cardiovascular system 76–9
carrier oils 11
castration 112
cataract 71, 80
chest compression 53
chest pain 75
cheyletiella 115
Chinese medicine 29–30
chiropractic 36
chlorella 47–8
choosing a puppy 120
chorea 93, 118
circulation see cardiovascular system
cirrhosis 100
clearing the airway 53
cod-liver oil 47
colic 99
colitis 6, 102
collapse and shock 57
colour therapy 31–2
commercial dog foods 41–2
common diseases and conditions 50–125
congestion 77
conjunctivitis 68–9, 71, 72, 118
constipation 93, 101
convulsions 91, 92, 108, 118
coprophagia 124
corneal ulceration 70, 71, 72

coughing 73, 74, 76, 96, 118, 119
Cushing's disease 82
crystals and gems 32–3
cystitis 103, 105
cyst, salivary 94

dandruff 61
decoctions, making 18
defecation
  frequent 102
  straining 99, 101, 102, 111
dehydration 104–5, 118
depression 48, 106
dermatitis 6; see also eczema
dermatophytosis see ringworm
diabetes mellitus 71, 80–1, 91, 100, 102
diarrhoea 20, 82, 99, 100, 118, 119
diet see nutrition
  changes in 45
  home-made 43–4, 46
  incorrect 63, 87, 90
  vegetarian 43
diffuser, using a 10, 11
digestive disorders 10, 19
digestive system 94–102, 118, 119
discharge 40
  ear 66
  eye 68–9, 70
  nasal 74, 118, 119
  vaginal 107
disc protrusion 87–8
dislocation
  of joint 86
  of patella 86
distemper 91, 93, 118
dowsing 37
drinking water 39
drooling 94, 95
dropsy see ascites
drugs, conventional 6, 17, 51, 70
  use of natural medicines with 9, 76
  reaction to 57
'dry eye' see kerato conjunctivitis sicca
dystocia 109

ear flap, swollen 67
ear mites 66, 116
ears and eyes 66–72
ear-scratching 66, 116
eclampsia 108

eczema 38, 39
  acute 60–1
  chronic 6, 62
electro-crystal therapy 33–4
electro-magnetic fields 39
emergencies 52–9
emotional disorders 14, 21, 22, 23
encephalitis 92
endocrine system 80–2
energy flows 24, 26
energy, lack of 77
entropion 68, 70, 71
environment 7, 38–40
epilepsy 91
epiphora 72
epistaxis 75, 118
essential oils 9, 10–12
exercise 40, 76, 87
eye drops, administering 69
eyesight 47

faeces
  blood/mucus in 102
  -eating 124
  lack of 101
falling 91
false pregnancy 106, 107
feeding see nutrition
female reproductive system 106–10
fever 75, 90, 100, 107, 108, 118
first aid 53
fits see convulsions
fleas 40, 115, 117
flower essences 9, 21
flower therapies 30
foreign bodies 60, 65, 68, 73, 74, 75, 96, 97, 98
fractures see bone fracture

garlic 9, 15, 19, 48
gastric torsion 98
gem essences 9
gems 32–3
geopathic stress 40
gingivitis 95
glands
  adrenal 82
  anal 63
  enlarged 80, 96
  lymph 79
  mammary 79, 106, 107
  thyroid 81
glaucoma 72
glucose, deficiency of 80, 108

grief 124
grooming 40
growth, rapid 90

haematoma 56, 67, 116
haemolytic disease 78
haemorrhaging 56, 67
Hahnemann, Dr Samuel 13
hair loss see alopecia
halitosis 94, 95
head-shaking 66, 67, 68, 74, 116
healing 24, 34–5, 47
health-checks 40
health-food stores 11, 22
health supplements 47–8
healthy life 38–48
heart disease 57, 76, 119
heart massage 53
heartworms 117
heatstroke 59
herbal medicine 7, 9, 17–20
herbs, gathering and storing 18–19
hip dysplasia 87
homesickness 23, 124
homoeopathic remedies 9, 13, 126
  contamination of 15
  potency 14–15
homoeopathy 6, 7, 13–16
hookworms 117
hormones 9
  imbalance of 62, 106, 108, 109, 110
  reactions 46
humidifier 38
hunger, increased 80, 82
hygiene 40
hyperactivity 19, 48, 123
hypersexuality 112
hypothyroidism 81

immune system 10, 24, 47, 118
  disease of 6, 27, 38, 60, 62, 70, 83, 89, 95, 100
incontinence 89, 104, 105
infection 47, 60, 62, 64, 65, 74, 75, 79, 83, 89, 90, 92, 95, 97, 103, 107, 108, 112
  ear 66–7
  eye 68–9, 71, 72
  specific 118–19
infertility 108, 118

inflammation
  brain tissue 92
  ear 66
  eye 68, 71
  gum 95
  joint 83
  mouth lining 95
  nerve 92
  pancreas 100
  prostate gland 111
  testicles 112
infusions, making 18
insulin 82, 83
intestines
  disorders 98, 99
  worms 117
intussusception 99
ionizers 38, 39
iridology 35
irritability 21
itching 60, 62, 63, 91,
  114, 115, 116
  of ears 66, 68, 116
  of eyes 68–9

joint dislocation 86
joints see musculo-
  skeletal system

kelp 46
'kennel cough' 73, 118
kerato conjunctivitis sicca
  70
kidney disease 83, 95,
  97, 104, 118

lameness 85, 86, 90, 118
land 39–40
laser treatment 26
lethargy 81, 82, 100
lice 115
lifestyle 40
ligaments see musculo-
  skeletal system
limbs, twitching of 93
liver disease 76, 77, 97,
  100, 118
lungworms 73
lyme disease 118
lymphadenopathy 79
lymphoma 79; see also
  cancer

magnetic fields 15
male reproductive
  system 111–12
mammary glands 79,
  106, 107
massage 10, 11
mastitis 107, 110
melanomas 113
meningitis 92
mental disorders 14, 21,
  22, 23

meridians 24, 26
metabolism 10, 46, 48
  disorders of 91
metritis 107
'milk fever' see eclampsia
milk production 110
  lack of 110
minor therapies 7, 28–37
mites 115, 116
motion sickness see
  travel sickness
mouth ulcers 95, 118
moxibustion 25
muscle
  stiffness 119
  stretching and
  weakness 82
  swelling 89
  tremors 82, 91, 108
  twitching 93
  wastage 89
musculo-skeletal system
  24, 83–90, 118
muzzle, using a 53
myositis 89

nasal discharge 72, 118,
  119
natural therapies 7, 8–37
neosporosis 119
nerves 88, 90
  degeneration of 89
nervousness 23, 48, 121
nervous system 24,
  91–3, 119
neuritis 92
nosebleeds see epistaxis
nutrition 7, 41–5
nutritional supplements
  46–7

obesity 45, 81, 103, 108
odour (at ear) 66
oedema 76, 77, 104
orchitis 112
osteoarthritis 84–5
osteochondrosis 90
osteomyelitis 90
osteopathy 36, 84
osteosarcoma 113
otitis externa 66–7
otitis media 116
  and interna 68
overdosing 9, 19

pancreatic disease 82, 97
pancreatitis 100
paralysis 24, 87, 88, 118
parasites 40, 48, 60,
  66–7, 73, 78, 101,
  115–17, 118
pharmacies 11
pharyngitis 96
phosphorus 16

photophobia 72
physiotherapy 35
phytotherapy see herbal
  medicine
pining 124
plants 10, 13, 17, 18
pneumonia 74–5
poisoning 58, 71, 78, 91,
  93, 95, 96
pollution 9, 38, 46, 47
pregnancy 106–8, 109
prostatitis 111
pus 65, 90
pyloric stenosis 98
pyoderma 60–1
pyometra 107

radionics 37
red blood cells
  destruction of 118
  lack of 78
reflexology 31
relieving pain 10, 24, 26
reproductive system 118
  female 106–10
  male 111–12
Rescue Remedy 21, 22,
  57
respiratory disorders 10,
  12, 14, 19, 38
  congestion 74
  coughing 73, 74, 118
respiratory system 73–5,
  118
restlessness 91, 106
restraining a dog 53
ringworm 117
roundworms 117
royal jelly 48, 83

salivary cyst 94
salt 41
  reducing intake of 76
Schuessler, Dr William 28
seaweed 46
seborrhoea 62
sexual behaviour see
  hypersexuality
shock 79
  collapse and 57
side-effects 6, 17, 26
sinusitis 12, 26, 38, 74,
  118
skin 60–5
skin disorders 14, 26, 40;
  see also itching
  anal irritation 63
  condition 48
  infection 82, 117
  inflammation 60
  swelling 40, 65

skin tests 40
'slipped disc' see disc
  protrusion
smell, sense of 66
sneezing 74
sore throat 80, 96
spinal injury 87, 105
spondylosis 88
sprains and strains 85
steroids 9, 82
stiffness 25, 83–4
  hindleg 87, 118
  muscle 119
  spinal 88
stomach disorders 98
stomatitis 95
straining
  to defecate 99, 101,
  102
  to give birth 109
  to urinate 103
stress 102, 107, 123
stud tail 64
supplements 7, 46–8
swaying 89
swelling 60
  abdominal 76, 82, 106
  ear flap 67
  eye 72
  facial 95
  glandular 107
  limbs 77, 85, 86, 90
  muscle 89
  testicles 112

tablets 7, 14, 18, 22,
  48
  administering 15, 49
  contamination of 15,
  49
tapeworms 117
tear
  drainage 72
  production, deficiency
  in 70
teeth 40, 47, 94
tendons see musculo-
  skeletal system
testicles 118
  painful 112
tetanus 91, 119
thirst, increased 80, 82,
  104, 107, 118
thrombosis 82
ticks 115, 118
tourniquets 53
toxoplasmosis 80, 119
travel sickness 125
T-touch massage 30–1,
  83, 85
tumours 66, 68, 72, 73,
  74, 75, 77, 82, 92,
  101, 103, 104, 105,
  107, 112

ulcers
  corneal 70
  mouth 95, 118
urinary system 103–5
urination, frequent 103
urine
  blood in 103, 104, 111
  difficulty in passing 111
  leakage of 105
urolithiasis 104–5
uveitis 72

vaginal discharge 107
vegetarian diet 43
vets, seeking assistance
  from 7, 9, 51
visual impairment 71
vitamin A 88
  and D 47
vitamin C 46
vitamin E 47
vomiting 82, 97, 98, 99,
  100, 104, 118
  inducing 58
  projectile 98

warts 64
  covering 64
water, drinking 39, 41
weakness 78, 82, 87, 118
weight control 45, 76
weight loss 77, 81, 83,
  100, 104, 119
whipworms 117
wild animals 17, 43
worms 99, 117
wounds 54–5, 92
  wrapping 55

yeast 46